GOD'S PRESCRIPTION
FOR PERSEVERING

PAIN

THE PLIGHT OF FALLEN MAN

DR. JIM HALLA

AMBASSADOR INTERNATIONAL
GREENVILLE, SOUTH CAROLINA & BELFAST, NORTHERN IRELAND

www.ambassador-international.com

Pain

The Plight of Fallen Man

Second Edition

© 2019 by Dr. Jim Halla

ISBN: 978-1-62020-906-6

eISBN: 978-1-62020-919-6

Cover Design and Page Layout by Hannah Nichols
Ebook Conversion by Anna Riebe Raats

AMBASSADOR INTERNATIONAL
411 University Ridge Suite B14
Greenville, SC 29609, USA
www.ambassador-international.com

AMBASSADOR BOOKS
The Mount
2 Woodstock Link
Belfast, BT6 8DD, Northern Ireland, UK
www.ambassador-international.com

The colophon is a trademark of Ambassador, a Christian publishing company

Contents

INTRODUCTION

PAIN IS NOTHING NEW. EVERYONE experiences it at some time in his life. Many people are writing about it. If you search various resources, as I did, you will find proliferation, not consensus, in terms of what pain is, its significance, and how you should approach it. So why another book on the subject? Good question. Let me tell you where I am coming from and then you decide for yourself.

When there is proliferation and no consensus, you need to ask why. There seem to be two possible answers: either everything "works" and pragmatism rules the day ("If it *works* use it.") or nothing works and everyone is simply giving his "best shot." If everything works, then you really don't need to read any further. Your solution is just as valid as the next person's. If everything works, I wonder why so many people continue to come to my office seeking help.

On the other hand, if nothing works (which is probably why you decided to pick up this book), then you are probably open to consider what I have to say. However, my intent is not to offer just one more opinion. I intend to challenge your thinking, excite your motivation, and change the way you approach the subject of pain.

I have been observing and caring for patients with complaints about pain for several decades. I diligently applied various approaches in an effort to help these hurting patients. The results were disappointing, both for me and the patients. Based on what people have told me and on my evaluation of the results using these various approaches, I concluded that there must be a better way, a superior answer to the fact that pain is a problem. Having found it, my challenge then became: How do I present this far superior approach to pain?

As a rheumatologist, I see patients daily who tell me about their struggles. They have an overwhelming desire for relief. They often did the best they could. They worked hard at what they thought was best for them. But they were disappointed in and with their situation. They had a body they did not like and pain that they had no use for. I tried to help them, but we both were swimming in a sea of various approaches to pain relief! And it seemed as if we were both drowning. Oh, some patients appreciated my efforts and even told me they were better and the treatment was working.

But then I became increasingly aware of what "better" and "works" were all about. I realized that pain is subjective and personal. Only the sufferer himself knows about it. It can't be measured. That was a major insight. It also became clear that pain was a given in the world in which we live. So putting those two things together, I began to write down things that challenged the patient's thinking and desires. Over time and with the help of my patients, I formulated a series of "Pain Papers" (see page 215 for more information). I use these in the office today as I treat patients with what I believe is a far superior approach to the problem of pain.

I have written this book in order to challenge your thinking, excite your motivation, and change the way you approach bodily problems. I have included a chapter on the anatomy and physiology of the pain system which I have attempted to make medically correct but "user friendly." In that chapter, I have drawn certain important conclusions based on the design of the body and how it functions.

Chapters 3-7 present the "majority opinion" regarding pain and what others believe should be done about it. I call that opinion "the wisdom of the culture." The proliferation of material that one sees is a reflection of that wisdom. I challenge you now, and throughout the first seven chapters, in regard to this wisdom: Is it wisdom or not? To answer that question, ask yourself: What is the result of the culture's approach to pain and pain relief? As I have cared for patients, they have given me a clear answer. I have recorded the results of following the culture's wisdom in chapters 5 and 7.

By the time you have read through chapter 7, you should be with me in terms of the results of the proliferation and application of the culture's answer to pain and the hope of pain relief. I will give you a sneak preview: the wisdom of the culture results in just the opposite of what patients are looking for. Now you are ready for the superior answer to the problem of pain and desire for pain relief. This is presented in chapters 8-10. These chapters contain the good news. The good news always comes on the heels of the bad news, but knowing the bad news is one way we understand that the good news is good. I progressively open up the beauty of that superior answer in those three chapters and put it all together in chapter 11.

CHAPTER ONE

PAIN: ITS FREQUENCY, PREVALENCE, AND IMPLICATIONS

A PATIENT COMES TO THE office with the following complaints as she slowly climbs onto the examining table: "I am stiff for hours in the morning, hardly able to get out of bed, I hurt all over, I am having difficulty getting done what I need to get done." She has tender, swollen joints and reduced mobility and function. She is quite discouraged. This thirty-five-year-old mother of three, previously in good health, has *rheumatoid arthritis* (RA). Her pain and stiffness are new experiences for her. She asks with an irritated, anguished look: "What can be done? I am only 35 years old and have a lot to do. Will this be with me and bother me the rest of my life?" What if the answers to those questions are less than what she hopes for, wants, and expects? Pain and fatigue seem to be her constant companions. They intertwine with her responses of anger, fear, anxiety, discouragement, and self-pity. These responses, however, only aggravate the pain.

Another woman, 29 years of age, visits her physician and reports that she has had pain "all over" for her entire life. She has never worked and reports that she cannot work because of her life-dominating pain. As the physician listens to the story, he is struck by the fact that pain seems to control her life: she marches to the drumbeat of her pain. She reports that pain is her constant companion. It is there when she awakens, through the day, and when she retires at night. Nights are often unpleasant because her sleep is restless. As she describes it, tomorrow usually brings nothing different. Upon physical examination, she has no joint swelling, her muscle strength is normal, and her range of motion is normal is all of her joints. However, the patient bitterly complains of pain especially when the physician moves her joints. When her physician presses and pushes along the spinal muscles of her back and neck, she reports pain at specific areas. She is diagnosed as having *fibromyalgia* (FM).

These patients are typical of patients seen in the office of a rheumatologist and have two things in common: pain and the desire to get rid of it. They have been labeled as having chronic pain and have identified themselves as pain sufferers. Because of what they think about the pain and what is causing it, each has established a strategy or an agenda for their lives. This plan includes hopes and expectations. Each vigorously pursues her agenda, which usually includes finding a cause for the pain that can be treated with removal of the pain. The purpose is to feel and function better. Most patients build their lives around the relief of pain or learning how to live with it. The latter is rarely defined.

While you may not have been diagnosed as having RA or FM or any of the other hundred or so musculoskeletal conditions (this includes problems of the bone and joint-arthritis, as well as problems of soft tissue including tendon, bursa, muscle, and ligaments), at some point in life you will encounter pain of some type for various reasons and for a varying duration. The reason: pain is universal. Pain is a reality in our world and in our bodies. Pain has been present since the fall of Adam and Eve (Genesis 3:15–17), and it has left its trail through time.

To get a grasp on the magnitude of this problem, I searched various sources. The presence and, therefore, the problem of pain is attested to by statistics from many sources. A good place to start was with the Internet. When I went on line in October 2000, using Alta Vista as the search engine, I pulled up 87,360 sites related to pain, 68,151 related to pain relief, and 8,631 related to pain treatment! When I requested chronic pain, 1,780 sites appeared. A comparison with other search titles included: cancer (2,186,630), cancer treatment (64,458), cardiovascular disease (79,622), heart disease (7,440), RA (1,805), and FM (3,495). It seems that everybody is writing about pain!

The subject matter varied and included advertisements for pain clinics, personal statements regarding pain and painful conditions, different modalities of treatments such as exercise, alternative medicine, nutrition, magnets, home remedies, mind over matter, nature, music, and other nonmedical treatments.

Thus, as the numbers attest, there is proliferation in this area. This would suggest that either everything works and everybody has the answer or nothing works and nobody has the answer. Yet some people obviously think their answer is *the* answer or at least *an* answer. The only consensus seems to be that pain is a reality and a problem in the world in which we live, and relief is essential at all costs. In contrast, the problem is that there is no consensus on what to do about it or how to obtain pain relief.

Figures from the medical literature are just as compelling. Pain is the primary presenting symptom in over 80% of physician visits per year, and almost 20% of the patients describe their pain as unrelenting and severe.[1] Another estimate is that between 15 and 20% of the population in industrialized countries describe themselves as having pain that is acute; between 25 and 30% describe themselves as having chronic pain. The cost of treatment exceeds 80 billion dollars per year in the United States alone.[2] (The terms *acute* and *chronic* are defined in chapter 2) Almost half of all Americans will seek some type of treatment for pain yearly.[3]

According to a 1996 telephone survey, "46% of respondents experienced severe pain at some time in their lives with nearly one-half of these episodes attributed to chronic backaches and one third to 'arthritis.'"[4] In the United States alone, between 50 and 75 million people have some form of recurrent or persistent pain.[5] This makes pain the single most common reason that compels patients to seek medical and dental help.

When considering specific areas of the body, it has been estimated that of the one-half of Americans who seek medical help for pain yearly, seven million complain of newly diagnosed back pain.[6] In fact, lower back pain is reported to rank second next to the "cold" as the most common affliction of mankind.[7] Over 65% of those studied have reported back pain at some time during their lives. Further, it is estimated that 15 to 20% of the population in the United States has back pain in any one year.[8] Neck pain, while a common complaint, is reported less frequently than lower back pain. Still neck pain and stiffness are reported in 30 to 50% of patients in one study.[9]

Pain is the most common symptom in rheumatic musculoskeletal conditions and diseases. These disorders (which include soft tissue rheumatism such as FM, bursitis, and tendinitis and those such as RA, osteoarthritis, and gout; and connective tissue diseases such as *systemic lupus erythematosus*) are among the most frequent medical conditions seen by physicians, with about 30 million Americans diagnosed as having one of them.[10] The prevalence increases with age and in certain occupations. In addition, statistics confirm that musculoskeletal conditions rank first in the frequency of physician visits, second in frequency of hospitalization, and fourth in frequency of conditions requiring surgery that is performed in hospitals.[11]

Finally, when considering nonrheumatic conditions, approximately 70% of patients with cancer report moderate to severe pain during the course of their illness, and 20 to 50% are experiencing pain at the time of diagnosis.[12] Other chronic pain conditions include nerve damage from any cause such as diabetic neuropathy and neuralgia of all types, sickle cell disease, endometriosis, and headache.[13] Few are spared the experience of headaches at some time during their lifetime, and "severe, disabling headaches are reported to occur at least annually by 40% of individuals worldwide."[14]

Truly, pain is a reality. The statistical data, as well as my personal experience, confirm that many people complain of pain and have been labeled as pain-sufferers. So what should a person think and do? How should he respond? Does his response have anything to do with pain's origin, intensity, and duration? Where should he turn for answers? To the medical community? To contemporary wisdom? To alternative medicine? To a combination of all the above? To the Bible? Does the Bible have answers? If the Bible has answers, do they focus on relief or how to live when there is no relief in sight? Are the Bible's answers significant and are they sufficient for a person's daily life when he is faced with a body that hurts, sometimes with no prospect for relief? Is it possible that the Bible's answers are not only sufficient but superior to anything that today's society can provide?

Together, we will attempt to answer all those questions and even more. What follows is the product of what I do every day as a physician, caring for patients who are real people with real-life problems. Patients are not simply chart numbers or problems with legs. So I begin my care of a patient by getting to know the person: his hopes, fears, expectations, wants, and desires. After taking his history, completing a physical examination in the office, and reviewing x-rays and laboratory data, I am in a position to begin to discuss the results of my findings. Once a diagnosis is made, it is also important to teach him about that diagnosis. Part of that teaching includes helping the person understand the body he has, how it has been designed, and how it usually functions. In the next chapter, we will answer the questions of why there is pain, what the source of the pain is, how it gets to the brain, and how the brain knows it is pain.

CHAPTER TWO

THE PAIN SYSTEM: ITS ANATOMY AND SIGNIFICANCE

SINCE PAIN IS PHYSICAL BODILY discomfort, it is appropriate to study the body and the system that carries pain messages from the periphery of the body[a] to the spinal cord and then to the brain for evaluation and interpretation. Since the body and its various systems are designed to function purposefully, pain can serve as a warning system, an attention-getter, much like the light on the dashboard of a car. It tells you that something is wrong. It is designed to be unpleasant in order to get your attention.

Given the complexity of the pain system and general lack of knowledge and familiarity with it, why should you and I study it? I chose to discuss it here because knowing the body and understanding the "ins and outs" of this system have proven beneficial to my patients. After I have taught them, patients have told me that they appreciate "somebody caring enough to educate me on how my body is designed to work." The idea that somebody takes time to help them learn about their bodies is comforting and leads to hope and confidence. It also

---

a   The "periphery" is the general term for parts of the body that are not central and includes such parts as the skin, muscle, tendon, ligament, bone, joint, and soft tissue around the bone and joint. It also includes the protective lining or membrane around internal organs of the body such as the liver, spleen, lung, and heart. Pain receptors in these areas send pain signals to the central portion of the body: the spinal cord and brain.

makes it easier to present proper treatment options to them. I hope you will have the same response!

Proper understanding helps remove doubts and fear of the unknown, both of which can arouse responses that intensify symptoms. With proper understanding, the patient is able to function more efficiently by avoiding that which aggravates his problem and by continuing that which is potentially helpful even if there is some pain. The reality of the situation is that the pain he is experiencing, what causes it, and his response to it are crucial to what he hopes, wants, fears, expects, or desires to happen. Knowledge is important in overcoming bodily problems daily. Without correct facts, false ideas will affect the person's wanting and thinking. Acting according to those facts result in aggravating and worsening pain.

A basic, obvious principle regarding pain is that it is felt or perceived. Since this is true, pain is clearly sensory. Pain, as a sensation, is the conscious awareness of a certain stimulus. How is pain felt or sensed?[a] The feeling of pain occurs in the body, first in that part of the body called the periphery. Some call this sensation the *announcement* of pain.

In an effort to simplify the anatomic pathways and the process of pain transmission,[b] consider a word picture.[15] Picture the pain signal

---

a   I use the word *feel* to describe sense perceptions. A person senses, feels, or experiences pain. By definition, this is the ability of the nerve endings and nerves to sense the stimulus, and the brain's function to perceive, interpret, and evaluate the pain impulses and react to them. In addition, I use the word *feeling* in two ways. First, I use it to describe sense perceptions when I am referring to pain. Pain is defined as a bodily physical discomfort. Second, I use it to describe the feeling state related more to one's thinking as he describes how he "feels." Some would refer to these feeling states as emotional states or emotions. In contrast to emotions, pain has discrete anatomic pathways that move the pain signal from the periphery to the brain. Emotions are God-given and are designed to motivate in order to get something done. They are generally defined as positive or negative feelings with mental and physical manifestations in the body. All emotions indicate something you do as a whole person. For example, people may speak of "being angry" or "feeling angry." The truth is that the person is angry. See David Powlison: "What do you feel?" The *Journal of Pastoral Practice*, 1992; 10:50–61.

b   This process is called *nociception*, which is the neurochemical process by which a pain as a small object that is constantly in motion along a pathway or roadway. The pain signal is picked up by a pain receptor (starting point or nociceptor) at the end of a nerve fiber (the road) that is connected to the spinal cord. The pain receptor is a special nerve ending that can sense unpleasant stimuli such as a cut, burn, or heavy pressure.

The impulse travels along the nerve, encountering junctions (synapses) that must be crossed to reach the spinal cord. Chemicals that are released from cells help or hinder the crossing of the pain impulse. The signal may meet resistance at the junctions and at the spinal cord. This resistance is a good thing because otherwise too many pain signals could reach the brain resulting in sensory overload.

Once the pain message enters the spinal cord, it is transmitted through a group of interconnected nerve cells (in an area of the spinal cord called the dorsal horn) to reach nerve pathways in the spinal cord that carry the signal upward to the brain. The impulse is further monitored as it crosses junctions to reach higher centers of the brain, where the impulse is evaluated and interpreted. Therefore, pain is felt in the central nervous system (CNS; see footnote a, page 23), first in the part of the brain called the thalamus and then in higher pain centers.

At the same time, the pain message may be inhibited by the brain. There are descending nerve fibers from the brain to the spinal cord toward the initial point of entry of the pain impulse.[a] These fibers can serve to reduce the transfer of pain signals to the brain through the

---

signal is carried or transmitted from the periphery to the central nervous system (CNS).
a   These fibers are known as descending pain inhibitory fibers. They regulate the transfer of nociceptive signals by the spinal nerve cells and fibers to the higher brain centers. These fibers receive sensory input from various brain sites, in particular the brainstem: midbrain, pons, and medulla. Upon electrical stimulation of these areas of the brainstem, these systems can modify pain sensation resulting in less pain (analgesia). Reactions to other painful stimuli are, therefore, inhibited. They form endogenous antinociceptive systems (EANS) which are internal anti-pain systems. These EANS can be activated by numerous stimuli including pain itself, illness, and conscious thought.

release of various chemicals, thereby decreasing the number of pain signals that reach it. Thus, the point of entry of the pain signal into the spinal cord from the periphery receives not only the pain signal from the periphery but signals from nerve fibers that descend from the brain.

The pain system, then, is programmed as a two-way system to regulate pain by increasing and decreasing pain signals that reach the brain. Pain regulation is done by ascending nerve fibers that carry pain signals *up* to the brain from the point of entry of the pain signal into the spinal cord, and nerve fibers traveling *down* from the brain to reduce pain signals that are able to leave a specific area of the spinal cord (specifically, the dorsal horn) to reach the brain.

The body has its own pain killers and pain enhancers. Cells in the brain and spinal cord produce chemicals that are similar to morphine. These chemicals reduce pain in the same way that morphine, a narcotic drug, does. The body produces them as a pain reliever. Two of these pain-regulating chemicals are endorphin and enkephalin. They may be released in response to pain itself, exercise, acupuncture, and even a placebo. Other substances (such as substance P) in the body do just the opposite: they intensify pain. These stimulate nerve endings or activate normally silent nerve fibers, thereby increasing pain signals. These two systems work together creating a proper balance, functioning to protect the body so that pain is not eliminated but is moderated and directed.

So how does a person feel or sense pain? Where does pain come from? Think of pain and the pain signal as electricity going through a wire or even water going through a pipe. Pain is electrical and chemical energy in motion. It results from a series of electrical and chemical transfers of pain signals that move from a receptor to the spinal cord by nerve fibers and then to the brain.

How do these structures relate to each other? Pain is perceived or felt in various areas of the body when pain receptors are stimulated or activated. These receptors, which are located on the end of nerve fibers, sense an unpleasant stimulus such as a cut, burn, or heavy pressure. Once the receptors are stimulated, a series of impulses (or signals) are set in motion and travel to the spinal cord by nerve fibers that are connected to the pain receptor. These receptors are of different types and respond to different types of stimuli (such as touch, pressure, warmth, and heat). The speed at which pain impulses travel along the nerve fiber varies depending on many factors (such as the diameter of the nerve fiber or whether the fiber is covered with a myelin sheath).

Once they reach the spinal cord, the impulses meet nerve cells that are able to function as gatekeepers, allowing or refusing to allow the pain impulse to pass to the brain. After entering the spinal cord, the pain impulse travels in nerve fiber bundles upward toward the brain. Other parts of the nervous system are stimulated into action so that bodily movements occur to reduce or eliminate the unpleasant sensation that triggered the message.

For example, when someone places his hand in the way of a saw blade and is cut, he immediately removes it. In addition, within the spinal cord, the message may be changed so that it is toned down. This happens when a person rubs, massages, or applies pressure to the injured area. Nerve cells in the spinal cord release chemicals that may increase or decrease the passage of nerve impulses to higher centers of the brain.

In the brain, the impulses first arrive in the thalamus, which is a sorting and switching station for pain impulses. The thalamus, upon receiving the impulses, quickly sends them to other parts of the brain (the cerebral cortex, including the frontal lobes, and limbic system) for evaluation and interpretation. Nerve input from the cerebral cortex contributes to pain perception in such a way that a person's attitude and thinking influence the perception of the pain signal (the cerebral cortex is involved in various cognitive activities including intelligence and thinking). The limbic system is not a separate system a collection of structures with a variety of functions that supports of bodily function. It is the portion of the brain that deals with several key functions: emotions, motivations, memories, learning, and arousal (or stimulation). It operates by influencing the autonomic nervous system and the endocrine system. This design helps understand how feeling states (some would call them emotions see footnote a, page 18) such as anger, bitterness, and worry can worsen pain. It also helps explain how various sensations such as palpitations, rapid heart rate, abdominal discomfort with or without diarrhea, or sweaty plans) accompany complaints of pain.

By virtue of God's design of human anatomy, there is truth in the statement "the pain is in your head." This doesn't mean that you or any person doesn't sense pain or that pain is imagined. Rather, rightly understood, the statement means that the brain contributes significantly to how a person feels pain. Since God made man a duplex being (a twofold being and unit body and spirit), a person thinks in both his brain – outer man and he thinks in his heart his heart - his inner man. A study of human anatomy does not completely account for the link between thinking, wanting, and feeling (so-called emotions). Only a proper view of man which is found only in the Bible helps us to properly understand wanting, thinking, feeling, and doing. I expand on this concept later in the book. Said another way, "pain is in your head" means that although pain is physical and therefore felt in the body, what is in your head (body) and your heart (inner man) has much to do with how you sense pain. Since pain is perceived and felt, only you, the person who feels the pain, know its presence, extent, and intensity.

However, responses to pain in terms of what a person says and does can be measured to some extent. A person's thinking can even be measured. How? You ask him what he is thinking and wanting and how each relates to pain—feeling. A person's thinking about himself, about life which is actually God's providence, pain, and his condition and what he thinks is causing pain, will have a significant influence on the intensity and severity of his pain.

This leads to another essential principle of pain: since pain is a sensation and is felt, the perception of pain can be changed. Pain perception is modifiable. And because the perception of pain can be changed, pain intensity may be increased or decreased. This principle follows from, as well as contributes to, how a person feels or senses pain.

There are many places in the pain system where modification of the pain signal may occur. These include the nerve receptor, the peripheral nerve, the spinal cord, and the brain. Various methods are used to eliminate the pain signal or to change the way a person perceives and feels pain. Pain medication of varying types work in the brain and spinal cord. Nonsteroidal anti-inflammatory medications work in the periphery.

There are other ways to change the perception of pain that are not dependent on things done to the body but come from within. Because there is a connection between a person's thinking, wanting, and attitude and his body, what one thinks influences pain perception. The brain activity does influence the health of the body and sensations in the body. This means that how and what a person thinks affects how he feels and interprets pain. What a person thinks about pain and the condition he has are crucial ingredients; for example, focusing on pain and pain relief only intensifies pain.[a]

In addition, what a person wants, desires, expects, and hopes for, affects his perception of pain and strongly influences his thinking. Sadness, discouragement, resentment, discontentment, and hopelessness can make pain worse, even intolerable. The opposite is also true: the absence of these and the presence of so-called positive attitudes can lessen pain and make it tolerable (see chapters 3 and 4).

The terms *acute* and *chronic* pain are arbitrary terms based on a person's description of the duration of the pain. Acute pain is generally thought to represent an initial response to tissue damage. The word acute comes from the Latin word meaning *needle*, referring to sharp pain of short duration.

On the other hand, chronic pain represents a sensation that is reported to persist beyond a certain period of time, including the time when an injury has been thought to have been healed. Chronic pain, then, describes pain that persists over a long period of time.

Acute pain is well defined with tissue injury followed by stimulation of pain receptors and subsequent transmission of the pain impulse to the spinal cord and then to the brain. People generally know and describe exactly where it hurts. The result of acute pain is muscle contraction and the activation of another system (the autonomic nervous

---

a   The term *focus* is used here to indicate a constant attention on pain, its consequences, and pain relief with the purpose of removing oneself from the discomfort, in the present as well as in the future. Terms to describe this kind of focus include: inappropriate, inordinate, and constant. There is an appropriate focus as well. This focus would fall under the guidelines of good stewardship of the body so that taking care of the body, not pain relief at all cost, is the motivating principle.

system[a] which controls such bodily functions as breathing, heart rate, and sweating, all of which can be measured).

In contrast to patients reporting acute pain, those who report chronic pain often have no observable tissue pathology, and if they do, the reported intensity of the pain is out of proportion to any tissue injury. People often speak of their pain as "hurting all over" or at least beyond the scope of the original injury or tissue pathology.[b] When people experience chronic pain, there is usually no initial activation of the autonomic nervous system. Therefore, the previously mentioned symptoms resulting from autonomic nervous system activation that often accompany acute pain, do not occur. This may help to explain why people with persistent (chronic) pain may not "look sick" or appear to be in pain when compared to people with acute tissue damage and injury.

Moreover, patients often report a more intense and exaggerated pain when there is a light touch or pressure or to the degree of tissue injury (or damage) identified. This means that the response of pain to light touch is out of proportion to what one would think the light touch should produce.[c] Unlike acute pain, the anatomy and physiology of chronic pain are poorly defined. Some researchers believe that chronic pain may be explained by aberrant central nervous system pain processing, hence the term "central" or "centralized" pain. "Central pain," also called "central sensitivity" or "centralized pain," is, therefore, the term

---

a   The nervous system of the body is composed of nerve cells and nerve fibers and is made up of the central nervous system (CNS), which includes the brain and spinal cord, and the peripheral nervous system (PNS), which extends from the spinal cord beginning at the anterior horn cell out to the periphery. There is a third system called the autonomic nervous system (ANS), which regulates normal body processes such as blood pressure, heart rate, breathing, digestion, perspiration, and sexual function.

b   The term given for this latter observation is *allodynia*. It is thought to be due to central sensitization which is thought to occur when there is hyperexcitability of CNS neurons.

c   The term given for this is *hyperalgesia*.

now now used to encompass any condition wherein pain is thought to be generated from the central, rather than the peripheral, nervous system. This concept highlights the contribution of thoughts and in regard to pain perception and its continuation. A number of reasons have been proposed to explain chronic pain, but all are inadequate. What is a common explanation in all of them is that thinking and attitude play a key role in its persistence, if not its initiation. This thinking and attitude are what many label a psychological factor.

Since the term *psychological* carries much baggage in our day and time, this area will be discussed in chapters 6 and 7. Suffice it to say that the term indicates that how a person thinks and acts is due to what has happened to him, whether it is from his circumstances, his genes, or his biology. In other words, he has no control or personal responsibility in responding to "what is out there." I don't use the term psychological because the term suggests a compartmentalization of the person and God is left out of the picture or He is only brought in as one of many forces and factors that bear on the person. It is also suggests that the person is a victim. A person's response to God's providence is affected by the person's view of God and self. God's providence is all that occurs in any person's life including pain. Nothing just is. Life does not have a life of its own or just is. Events and circumstances flow from God's control. The person is responsible for his responses to God and His control including the body that he has. All of these factors influence, don't cause, a person's response to them which affects pain perception. Since the person's response is related to his thoughts, desires, and attitude, pain perception can be changed. Therefore there is hope.

Let us look at a third principle concerning pain. Symptoms may occur because something is wrong with the body. Actual tissue damage or injury may be discovered or found. Because of this tissue damage, nerve signals are sent to the spinal cord and brain as previously described. However, a person may feel the same symptoms of pain when no discernible changes are found or discovered in the body. What is the explanation? It is always possible that there is undiscovered tissue pathology (damage, injury, or abnormality) due, in part, to the limitations of medical science. The body is not flawless and there will be many bodily symptoms for which a cause is never found.

A person may report symptoms even though there is no discoverable bodily problem. These symptoms may occur depending on how a person uses his body, including how he responds to *life* (God's providence) in general and bodily problems. One's response may include physical activity such as mowing the grass and cleaning the house. However, a person's thinking which is influenced by his wants, hopes, fears, and desires may produce symptoms – sensations that are felt, even measured in the body. Wanting and thinking not only drive bodily activity, but they influence bodily sensations. Therefore, in those situations where no discoverable bodily problems are found, often symptoms are felt in the body as the result of a person's wanting and thinking.

People usually refer to symptoms without discoverable bodily abnormalities as stress and report that "stress made me hurt." In truth, it is a person's unbiblical response to life events (God's providence) that produces change in the body. This wrong way of thinking and wanting produces feelings inside his body as he processes what is happening outside of him. Pressure is what is going on outside of a person. Bad feelings are what a person produces inside by the way he thinks and reacts to things such as having pain and a body he doesn't want. This subject is taken up in greater detail in chapter 4.

Having reviewed the anatomy and physiology of the pain system (how the body's pain system works), I discussed certain principles of pain. Are you familiar and even comfortable with them? These included:

1. Pain is bodily physical discomfort and is perceived as an unpleasant sensation.

2. Since the perception of pain is changeable and modifiable, the sensation of pain is changeable. This is dependent on what and how a person thinks, which is determined in part by what they want and hope for. Ways of thinking can increase or decrease pain.

3. Symptoms of pain and feeling bad may occur when no tissue pathology or injury is demonstrated.

4. Acute and chronic pain are arbitrary terms based on a person's description of the length of pain.

The next chapter begins to look at the person who has pain, his goals and fears, and how the principles that were discussed in this chapter apply.

CHAPTER THREE

THE RELATION BETWEEN PAIN AND THINKING

IN CHAPTER 1, I INTRODUCED you to two patients with medical conditions who reported pain as a significant part of their lives. They had several things in common. Not only did each complain of pain but she also desired pain relief. Each pleaded, "Help me get rid of my pain." The fact of pain and the desire for pain relief are not new: pain has been present since the fall of Adam and Eve. Pain is universal, and the goal of bringing relief occupies much of the attention, time, and money of both patients and physicians alike.

So given these facts, what is the issue? The issue is not the presence of absence of pain but how he will respond to his condition which includes pain. A response to them is a response to God. So let's look at some responses.

The most common response is the desire for pain relief. Pain gets one's attention By God's design, there was no pain pre-fall. Post-fall things changed. The nervous and pain systems that I described in chapter 2 became a both a blessing and a curse. Remember Genesis 3:16? God promised pain in childbirth for the woman. This is the first mention of the word pain in the Bible. However, it is not only the pain that should get attention but also what the person thinks the pain represents or may represent. Some common thoughts and concerns raised are: "What is causing this?" "Why do I hurt?" "What are the possible consequences of my pain and the bodily problem I have?" "How long will this go on?" "Can you help me control it?" "What about my lifestyle now that I have trouble doing things?" "This pain of mine makes me do things I don't like, especially when compared to the way I used to do things." Do these concerns sound familiar?

In order to dig deeper into the mindset and thinking that is motivating some patients who are seeking pain relief, let's look at a visit from Ms. Patient who is 30 years old and reports pain for the last ten years. Though not a real patient, she and her answers represent a composite of many patients I see. She may have any of the rheumatic conditions mentioned in chapter 1. So I ask her,

 —What is the problem?

 —I have this pain all over. I hurt when I do things, and I
 don't feel good.

 —How can I help?

 —I want to know why.

 —How would knowing "why" help?

 —We could find the cause of the pain and get rid of it or
 control it.

I wonder why that is so important to her, so I ask her, "Why? Help me understand what makes it so important." She answers . . .

 —I need to get rid of this pain because I have too much to do.
 People depend on me. I have no time for this pain and I am
 upset that I have it. I want to work and be useful, but I can't.

 —When you say you are "upset," what do you mean?

 —I mean I get angry and mad.

 —What are you angry about?

—Because I can't do things like I used to and I have to do
things like I don't want to. I want to be able to do things like
I used to and just lead a normal life. I just want to be me!

—What happens when you are thinking and wanting like that?

—The situation doesn't get any better and it may even get worse.

—When you say you "can't," do you mean you are paralyzed?

—No, but it feels like it. I don't like to move because it hurts.

—Are you telling me that "can't" really means "won't" and "don't"?

—Well . . . yes.

—And the reason you do this is in hopes of lessening your pain?

—Yes, and I want you to understand how bad I hurt. It's important to me for you to know.

—What makes it important?

—I am not sure.

—How would it help for me to know?

—I would know someone cared and would try to get me
relief. Nobody else has.

Ms. Patient has told me about her thinking, wants, fears, hopes, expectations, and goals. She has told me about her agenda to achieve them.
She finishes the interview by telling me, "I just want to feel better. I
don't need to hurt." She has no idea that she responding to God and
His control. She is in a theological battle.

This conversation is typical. It points out the fact that pain is not
an abstraction or simply an idea. It does not occur in a vacuum. Pain
and one's response to it are not neutral. Rather, the symptoms of pain
and bad feelings always occur in a real person with real problems who
thinks and feels a certain way. Pain, as does any circumstance and
situation, influences and stimulates a response but does not cause

the response. Influence is not the same as determines. Otherwise the person would be a victim. In addition to responding to pain, people respond to all the concerns and desires that flow out of those concerns including the desire for relief. They bring to the drawing board of life a plan (agenda) based on thoughts, wants, fears, hopes, and expectations. They have reached certain conclusions such as "pain is a bummer," "it's the pits," "it's hard." Because of these conclusions, they are trying to do something about it, even get rid of it, by finding someone or something that will help them. It is easy to respond to any situation without a proper vertical reference. Ms. Patient has shrunk her life so that it is personal and horizontal. If she moves vertically, toward God, there is a danger it is only to get relief.

Further, those who experience pain over a long period (chronic pain) begin to think a certain way. Often, they have been labeled and even label themselves as *chronic pain sufferers*. This label distinguishes them from those who experience pain of a much shorter duration. By the very nature of the definition, chronic pain persists, is harder to eliminate (otherwise, one would not be labeled a chronic pain sufferer), and attracts and occupies the attention of the patient and the medical profession alike. What is the importance of thinking of oneself as a chronic pain sufferer? A reference to two children's stories will help us in answering this question.

Do you remember the children's stories "The Ugly Duckling" and "Lambert the Sheepish Lion"?[16] In chapter 2, we learned that one's attitude and thinking affected how he perceived, felt, evaluated, and interpreted pain. Based on their perception of themselves, the swan and the lion, even though they had been what they were since birth, responded to their situations based on their perceptions. Thinking they were something else (the swan thought he was a duck and the lion thought he was a sheep), they tried to live as what they thought they were. However, reality finally set in and they changed. One day the ugly duckling, ridiculed all his life, looked at his reflection in the pond and saw not a duckling but a swan. He then lived his life as a swan. Lambert, encountering a wolf that threatened the flock, realized he was a lion, not a sheep, and acted accordingly. These two stories serve to emphasize that what a person thinks about himself influences how he thinks and acts.

An individual's choice of lifestyle is influenced by his perception of himself, of the body he now has, and of the potential consequences of each. Moreover, as I discuss in later chapters, a person's view of God is major determining factor of pain perception and his response to it. Usually he develops a plan – a strategy of "coping" – that includes any number of things, but especially some sort of pain relief. This may be the driving and motivating force in his life. He often builds his life around pain and pain relief.

As you recall from chapter 2, the physical discomfort of pain is felt in the body. The sensation of pain occurs at two places: in the body, away from the brain and spinal cord (called the periphery; footnote, page 17), and in the brain itself where the pain impulse must be recognized, interpreted, and evaluated. The person then hurts and feels bad. Pain should get the person's attention. At least it should remind the person of the fall and God's judgment but also God's grace. Pain then is a warning to alert man to be a good steward of his body.

As a result of the brain's interpretation and evaluation of the pain signal, the person may feel sad. Some call this an emotional response. If he frequently thinks about the pain in a certain way, such as not liking it very much and wanting it gone, the pain will be intensified (see footnote, page 22). This is part of the story of Ms. Patient.

Thus, there are two ways of "feeling" pain. One is the "feeling" triggered by the body as one senses pain outside the brain at the pain receptor level. The other is triggered by one's attitude and thinking after the pain impulse reaches the brain and is perceived (see footnote, page 22).

The simple fact is that you know that you have pain because you hurt. Fair enough. In addition, pain is like any other *symptom* such as fatigue, weakness, and even fear. A symptom is something experienced and subjective. It is known only because the person makes it known. It is reported by the patient and thus differs from a *sign*. A sign is something observed. It is an objective, demonstrated abnormality in and of the body.

For instance, a patient can report feeling feverish. That feeling is a symptom describing how he feels. Now, if one places a thermometer in his mouth and his temperature is 102°F, then he is not only reporting feverishness (a symptom), but he also has a sign – a fever that can be measured. But when we are talking about pain, there is no pain thermometer or pain gauge, only the person's report.

Pain, like any and all symptoms, is personal and subjective: only the person himself knows whether he hurts or doesn't hurt. If he reports "feeling fine" and has an elevated temperature (fever), then his report of feeling fine (a symptom of good feelings!) would be considered suspect and attention should be directed toward the sign and what it means. The above principle also applies if someone reports "no pain" but has evidence of a disease, especially if it is active (active RA for instance). The statement "no pain" should take a back seat to the issue at hand, which is the patient, his response, and his condition. So where should the physician place his emphasis? Should he decide not to treat because the patient reports no symptom of pain? Or should he treat the disease process? Because the patient has active disease, the decision to treat would be indicated regardless of the presence or absence of symptoms.

Since the pain impulse must be recognized, interpreted, and evaluated in the brain, and because of the connections within the brain that link thinking and feeling centers, it follows that attitude affects how one feels, interprets, and evaluates pain. That is, what someone thinks about his pain, the actual condition causing his bodily problems, and God's providence or God's control, influences how he feels and perceives pain. Further, what he wants, including pain relief, affects how he feels and perceives pain.

Our interview with Ms. Patient highlights these points. Ms. Patient clearly told me what she wanted from me: pain relief. She made no mention of her relationship with Jesus Christ. She told me about her thinking and wanting and how she had reached some important conclusions. This problem of pain was a "bummer" and now so was her life. She told me that the pain kept her from doing things she had to do and from helping people who depended on her.

She told me what she thought about her problem and herself (her identity): "I have no time for this pain" and "I want . . . to just lead a normal life." She told me what she expected of me: "I want to know why." "Can you find the cause of the pain and get rid of it" and "I want you to understand how bad I hurt."

Clearly from this you can see that the whole person is involved when it comes to pain and its perception. Therefore, the intensity of the pain can be changed by how one views pain. That is, by changing one's thinking and wanting regarding pain, he can feel more or less pain. Moreover, a person's view of himself, his bodily problems, and even life itself affect his perception of pain. But – and this is critical to understand – a person's perception of pain also influences his view of himself, his bodily problems, and life itself. It works both ways.

Here is an appropriate place to mention the terms *emotional* pain, *mental* pain, and *psychological* pain. These terms are usually contrasted with physical pain. They indicate hurting in the nonphysical realm and describe inner-man angst in its various forms. They describe how one feels and indirectly what one is thinking and wanting. Emotions however defined may be on display but emotions themselves don't hurt. Rather, sensations are felt in the body as one effect of an anger and fear. They allow for the compartmentalizing of the person as if there is more than one type of pain. However, by definition, pain is a physical bodily discomfort. It is physical and felt in the body. Moreover, pain is a whole person activity involving thinking and feeling. As we have seen, pain signals are sensed or felt in the periphery, carried to the spinal cord, and recognized in the brain. All of this occurs in the body. This means the pain signal is recognized, evaluated, and acted upon in the body. The individual will then respond both in his think-ing (mental activity) and feelings (he may feel sad or he may become angry: emotional response).

But as we have also seen, what a person is thinking and how he is feeling (sad, blue, discouraged, hopeless) affects his perception of pain. The result may be an intensification of pain. Based on these facts, it is accurate to speak of pain as *physical*. It is inaccurate to speak of pain in the nonphysical realm. Therefore, I do not recommend the use of the terms *emotional*, *mental*, or *psychological* to refer to pain.

A number of illustrations make the point regarding the connection between thinking, wanting, and how someone feels in his body. Picture a group of people sitting quietly visiting together. They hear a commotion from outside the room and investigate. Upon opening the door, they stand face to face with a large bear. What happens? Most people say they experience certain symptoms in their body: fast heart rate, faster breathing, skin changes, and fright. Yet none would be labeled as having heart or lung disease. No, the body, appropriately acting as it was designed, is responding to something outside of the person.

Now consider the same scenario, with a change – the bear is under the control of his trainer. These facts lead to changed thinking and wanting about the themselves and the situation and as a result changed feelings. Most would describe fewer symptoms and bad feelings. The presence of the trainer would reassure the people that the bear is not wild and this would change their thinking about the situation. As a result, there would be fewer symptoms. There is a connection between what one thinks and how one feels in his body. One's thinking, wanting, and attitude can be changed by something going on outside of one's self, which therefore leads to changed bodily feelings. People are not victims to that which is outside of them or to that which is inside of them. They can control thinking and wanting and changed feelings generally follow.

Consider another scenario: you receive a call from an Internal Revenue Service (IRS) representative who desires an appointment with you. No details are given. What happens? Your thoughts and expectations fly all about. You experience certain feelings, some considered bad. Your body responds to what you are thinking. Now, consider how different those feelings would be if the IRS agent told you the purpose for the meeting: to receive a refund rather than an audit!

An additional example involves a secretary. She works for a pleasant boss, but on this day she has been asked to meet a deadline requiring extensive typing. The boss asks her to skip breaks and eat lunch at her desk. He checks on her frequently. What could be going on with the secretary by the end of the day? It would not be surprising if she reports pain in her neck and shoulder areas. She meets her deadline and returns home only to feel continued pain well into the evening. Her muscles are tight and achy. If her neck and shoulder areas were examined, one might find firm areas or knots in her muscles. Where did those tight muscles come from? What's happening? The deadline has been met, the boss has gone, and yet she still feels pain in her body. Physically, she used her body in response to the increased work load. Could that be it? Possibly, but she also reports constant nagging thoughts of the day still bouncing around in her head. Prolonged tight muscles may be in response to the increased physical activity, but more likely they are due to her thinking about the day's work and about her desire to finish.

All of these examples share the fact that there is a relationship between things outside the person and his reaction and subsequent symptoms and feelings. This relation is by way of thinking, wanting, and perception. Symptoms and what one is feeling in his body may actually be precipitated by his thinking.

One final illustration, known as the placebo effect, drives home the relationship between thinking and the perception of pain. The term placebo usually refers to medications that are inactive and harmless. In the study of new drugs, patients are divided so that one group takes the study drug and the other a placebo. The effects of the drug are compared to those of the placebo. In most studies of rheumatic diseases, patients taking only the placebo report a 20 to 40% response rate in terms of improvement of RA. But the response usually is sustained no longer than one to three months. More recent studies in the treatment of RA do not include a true placebo group. It is considered unethical. In those earlier studies, the patients in the placebo group often reported improvement in their disease for one to three months but no longer. Various explanations are given for this, but the one most likely is the placebo's effect on the thinking rather than on the body.

Responses to pain may be controlled by the desire for pain relief, as is evident during my interview with Ms. Patient. Seeking pain relief was a driving force in her life. In addition, pain may be present when no actual tissue damage is found. Pain relief and avoidance of pain (even to the point of desiring that she had a different body than the one she is "stuck with") should not be the main goals in her life. If any of these are overriding goals, she will find herself in a cycle that I call the *boomerang effect*. Pain intensity increases as pain relief is not forthcoming. The greater the desire for pain relief, the greater the misery of pain and its intensity when that desire is not met. In other words, the more she wants the pain to stop, the harder it comes back on her. That is the boomerang effect.

Also, a response to pain is influenced by the belief that one's problem is different from everyone else's. Do you know of someone who thinks like that? He may conclude any number of things. For instance, he may think that his goal of treatment will never be reached. That seemed to be the case with Ms. Patient. Other conclusions that she could have reached include believing that improvement is impossible, that the difficulty is uncontrollable, and that no effective solution can be found. She has drawn conclusions about her situation: it is really bad.

What happens when Ms. Patient thinks this way? Based on her own experience and what she has been told or learned from other sources, she may focus on many things under one heading: pain relief. Often this focus is described as fearing the worst or worry or discouragement. She used the words upset and frustrated. She was not a happy camper. The more she desired to be pain-free or relatively free the more she hurt. Functionally, she told me that she was tied to her thoughts and demands including pain relief. Pain relief had become such a demand but she was unaware of it. She described the cycle as pain and more pain and she did not know what to do. Pain was a major complaint, regardless of whether or not the condition or disease could be controlled. The fact is: it is often hard, or even impossible, to control pain in this situation, and so the person may mistakenly conclude that worsening pain means worsening of his condition or disease.

What may happen? When I asked Ms. Patient to tell me about her day, she was more than willing to do so. This information helps me learn more about her and how her thinking and wanting affect her daily life.

—Please tell me about your day, from the time you awaken
  to the time you go to bed.
—I awaken with pain and go to bed with pain, but not every
  day. Some days are good days and others bad.
—What is a bad day and what determines that?
—Whether I hurt or not. I don't wake up and want to hurt.
  But when I feel pain, I go sit down, and if the pain doesn't
  get better, I lie down.
—What are you thinking then?

—I am thinking about wanting the pain to get better.

—And if doesn't?

—I just lie there hoping and waiting.

—For what?

—The pain to go away.

—And if it doesn't?

—I just hurt.

Ms. Patient is living life as a "couch potato," unwilling to do much because "it hurts too much." More time is spent in inactivity of the body and focusing on the pain and her undesirable situation. She knows and thinks it is bad and acts upon that belief. When she does become less active as a result of her view of the pain and bodily problems, the resulting condition is a *learned helplessness*. Her focused thinking and wanting was actually sinful. They influenced her feelings and the use or non-use of her body. A cycle of pain: discouragement, more discouragement, and finally hopelessness. Her view is that the situation will not improve. This hopeless way of thinking leads her to stop trying in the belief that she "can't." This cycle occurs because of wrong thinking and wanting and the results of acting on that thinking.

Ms. Patient's response to pain and bodily problems is also affected by her confidence and belief that she can act in a way so as to control her present and future destiny. Her hope is to lessen pain and control her condition or disease. If she is willing to pace herself during the activities of daily living, this produces confidence that "I can do it." On the other hand, when she is unwilling to "do" because of the pain (and as an attempt to avoid pain), she assumes the role of "couch potato." As she reported, her pain and bodily problems worsened. The net result was losing hope and confidence. People with less hope and less confidence usually complain of still more pain.

A patient's thinking in regard to hope, expectation, and the belief that something can be done for the condition or disease affects the intensity of pain. Ms. Patient lacked true hope. She had a *hopeso*. The object of her hopeso was a pain-free body. She did not know how to define biblical hope. Improved ability to be functional during pain and being satisfied with that improved function are not considered important to her. However, these are attainable, and if she focuses on these goals, her pain may actually be reduced.

On the other hand, I asked Ms. Patient about her good days:

—Those are the days I don't feel much pain – I don't hurt as much.

—What is happening in terms of thinking, wanting, and doing?

—I feel so good and remember how much I need to do and haven't done, so I go and do it even if it begins to hurt.

—What happens to the pain?

—I feel pretty good at first and then hurt more afterwards.

I call this the "road runner" approach to the problem of pain. Let me explain. The road runner is a person who is going, going, gone in terms of activity both mentally and physically. It is as if she is afraid to stop. "I feel good so I must accomplish all that I did not accomplish, want to accomplish, should accomplish, but may not accomplish" is her typical war cry. Doing, with or without pain as the goal of life, has replaced the goal of being pain free.

Such is Ms. Patient on her good days. However, there is a price to be paid in this approach to pain. Ignoring, even denying, that pain is present in the body she has and doesn't like usually results in increased pain. Ms. Patient told me that sometimes there is much pain during her tasks or after she completed her tasks. She was willing to put aside pain in order to accomplish what she thought was important.

A word about the stewardship of the body is in order. What does this mean? Simply put, stewardship is taking care of that which God has entrusted to you. Your body is the only one you will get in this life. Because everyone is a steward of his body, the question is "What type of steward are you: good or bad? Are you taking good care of the body God has entrusted to you or not?" However, taking care of the body (good stewardship) to promote good health or obtain pain relief can never be an end in itself. In fact, taking care of the body for the sole purpose of living longer, healthier, and more comfortably can become a preoccupation in and of itself. This, in turn, can lead to the pursuit of an agenda much like the relentless pursuit of pain relief.

So what is a person to do with and for his body? He should take care of it. The question is, "How?" From the previous discussions, it is apparent that stewardship is a Whole-person issue, just like pain. It includes both thinking, wanting, and doing.

Stewardship involves care of the inner and outer-man activities. It is logical and God-pleasing. Proper stewardship of one's body includes getting the facts about the physical problem, thinking correctly about them, and putting them into a biblical framework. It also requires getting the facts about the person himself. The good steward will apply those facts daily. He will be aware of the trio of thinking, wanting, and doing and their interrelationship with feelings.

Often a person will be tempted to focus on the way his life has changed, wishing for what he once had and becoming resentful about the body he now has. This change will be perceived as bad. This way

of thinking is an example of poor stewardship that affects the body:
how it feels and how it functions. Take Ms. Patient. Almost daily, she
compares how she is now (she has pain and a body that doesn't work
as she wants it to) with the way she used to be. This focus can only
aggravate her symptoms.

Consider these "ifs" in regard to Ms. Patient: If the hope is for a pain-
free body, and if the goal is pain relief and getting on with life, then
what is likely to happen? Usually, the result is more bodily problems
and pain.

So, as I continue to see Ms. Patient and get to know her, I will ask
her, "What is the likelihood of having a pain-free body now or in the
future?" I want her to think about the body as imperfect, flawed. Bodily
symptoms, including pain, are part of living in the world we do, with
the bodies we have. She answers something like this:

—"I know I hurt now and may do so for a long time, but I
hope that I can stop hurting. Anyway, I don't care about the
future, I only care about now."

In answer to my question of " . . . the likelihood of your having a
pain-free body . . . " Ms. Patient has missed the point. The reality of a
painfree body is virtually impossible in our fallen world (Romans 5:12-
14; 2 Corinthians 4:16-18). How Ms. Patient responds to that reality will
determine her perception of pain. An example of the principle of poor
stewardship of the whole person is the couch potato approach to life
mentioned previously, and evidenced by Ms. Patient. She does not like
what she has – a body that hurts; and does not like what she has lost –
her old lifestyle of doing and her previous body. The unmasked reality
she is faced is her dislike of God and His providence. She does not like
God. He has proven Himself untrustworthy because He has given her

this body and problem and He will not remove it. Not moving because "it hurts" only aggravates bodily problems and contributes to feeling more pain. She has let her feelings guide her and has accepted them as infallible. "No pain, no gain" has no place in Ms. Patient's vocabulary and thinking. Meeting personal responsibilities is delayed and even ignored. This seems to validate her predicament as hopeless and herself as helpless. She continues to spiral downward in this thinking and wanting, which results in further symptoms and bad feelings including more pain.

On the other hand, Ms. Patient once lived according to her feelings using the road runner approach to life. This seems far more acceptable to her and even pious to others. However, the body was not designed to function as a road runner. Patients who ignore pain in bursts of activity usually describe a significant increase in pain afterwards. This was the case with Ms. Patient. This leads to what I term the "yo-yo" (or "picket fence") syndrome because the person's activity level and pain level resemble the ups and downs of a yo-yo. She finds herself on a roller coaster as she acts on her feeling of pain or lack of pain in her body. This approach is rarely successful in achieving what is wanted: pain relief and getting things done with or without pain. That is because the body was never designed to be used this way. Doing things "for the sake of doing" as a lifestyle (or even for one day) is as elusive as the goal of having a pain-free body. Both are like the elusive "butterfly of love": a person has a hard time grabbing hold of them and gets tired in the trying, which only increases his misery. That was apparent as Ms. Patient told her story.

Both of these approaches ("couch potato" and "road runner") to pain and bodily problems are *guided and driven by feelings* which originate in and persists due to thinking and wanting in the whole person, her body and her inner man (the heart). Her thinking and wanting must change in both areas for her to victory. Victory is a term rarely used in this. I discuss this subject in latter chapters.. Rather, doing and not doing should be balanced and motivated by the desire to be functional given the body one has. This is good stewardship. Stewardship includes seeking pain relief but not as the primary goal in life. Stewardship also means doing, but again, not as the primary goal for life. Taking care of the body may result in pain relief or may not. No matter what kind of body a person has, or how it feels, he can always be more functional. That in itself brings satisfaction and contentment in life. Being satisfied in and with life changes one's perception of pain and often results in less pain.

Given the facts above, what is to be done when you are faced with the reality of living in a body you don't like for the rest of your life? You may well turn to the wisdom of the culture. What does contemporary medical science have to say? One area that needs discussion is depression and stress in connection with the management of pain. Is there a connection and if so what is it? This subject will be discussed in the next chapter.

CHAPTER FOUR

The Connection Between Depression, Stress, and Pain

WHEN I SEE PATIENTS, THEY tell me about pain, feeling bad, and hurting. Many of them, maybe like yourself, are concerned about how they feel and often wonder where these feelings come from. Pain tends to stimulate people to think and wonder. Here are some results of their thinking: "If I know the source of this pain and bad feelings, then something can be done to change them." "If these bad feelings are changed, then it is possible to have a body that is free, or almost free, of any unpleasantness."

These people are facing the fact that pain and feeling bad are an unavoidable part of life, and living in this fallen world demonstrates that. A concept that will be found repeatedly in this book is that to live wanting little or no unpleasantness is futile, even counterproductive and fits the term vanity of vanities by the author of the book of Ecclesiastes (1:9). Indeed, the pursuit of that goal usually results in greater pain. So if the pressures of life (actually God's providence) and stress (I will define this term later) influence a person to experience more pain, how do they do so? Is it the pressures of life that cause the pain or is it the way one responds to those pressures?

As we have seen in chapter 3, helping a person change his thinking and wanting enables him to respond differently to these pressures.

This often helps lessen pain. So a couple of questions before us are: How may a person respond, including thoughts, desires, and actions or inactions, to the pressures and trouble experienced in life, including bodily problems? Faced with pressure all around him, what will help him when he is feeling bad and suffering pain?

First, some facts and figures. Various sources report the presence and frequency of anxiety and depression, ranging from 25 to 70%, in various chronic conditions and diseases.[17] This has led some research-ers to conclude that the condition or the disease itself produces these feeling states, or that these feeling states are part of the condition.[18] However, the majority of patients with various rheumatic conditions and diseases are functional both at home and in the workplace. They do not become depressed, focus on pain and pain relief, or grumble and complain about their situation. What is the difference between the group with anxiety and depression and the group that is functional and not depressed?

During the time that I am with a patient, I gather information and collect data about what he wants and thinks. That is because (as we learned in chapters 2 and 3), patients come with a label and an idea of who they are or want to be (they have identified themselves). They come with fears, hopes, wants, expectations, and goals. These are all innerman or heart activities. They are accompanied by such terms as depression, fear, worry, anger, and being overwhelmed. The latter terms are rarely defined and when they are they so often fall under the rubric of emotions. However, when properly defined and unmasked, they are reactions to God and His control. At the core they are issues of control and resources. They have, and are developing, a plan to avoid pain. Symptoms such as pain and physical changes may occur as a result of pursuing those goals, hopes, and wants.

Often, I ask the patient for a list of factors that aggravate or bring about pain and bad feelings. More often than not, the patient will tell me: "Stress makes it worse." "When I get upset and discouraged then my pain gets worse." "Sometimes I just don't think I can go on and I sit down and have a pity party. I feel better for a little while but then it is back and I feel worse." "I try to do and function but it hurts and I want it to go away." "This pain really depresses me." "I know there must be something wrong in my body or I would not hurt like this."

When I ask the patient how pain depresses him, I often hear something like this: "I want to do and go but can't. I remember how I used to do things but now can't, and that makes me upset." Sometimes if I know the patient, I ask him: "What is it about the change in function that depresses you?" I will hear things such as "I don't want this pain" "I don't deserve this" "I have too many things I want to do and need to do and too many people depending on me."

Faced with these answers, there is further information I need if I am to best help my patient. I want to know such things as: How do you define depression? What is it about pain that causes depression? How do you define stress? What is it about that stress that causes pain? How do you respond to what is depressing you or causing stress? What is it about depression and stress that worsens or causes pain? How is this stress bad or unpleasant? What have been the results of your responses?

To begin with, an understanding of terms is in order. Keep in mind that both pain and bad feelings, from whatever cause, are symptoms and thus are personal and subjective. Remember chapters 2 and 3. In those chapters I distinguished between something wrong in the body and something wrong with the body. Symptoms are subjective, personal, and depend on the report of the person. Often they indicate something wrong in the body not necessarily wrong with the body. RA and cancer are examples of something wrong with the body. In addition, in chapter 2, I briefly introduced you to some things that produce symptoms. They may occur because some part of the body is damaged and not working right. To prove this requires tests by the physician. An abnormality may be identified by the doctor's physical examination, blood studies, or radiographic studies. Finding abnormalities may explain why pain is present.

However, the very same symptoms may be present when nothing causing them is discovered or found wrong in the body. The symptoms are actually present, but nothing shows up in the medical workup. The doctor cannot find anything in the body that accounts for the pain. This does not mean the symptoms are "in your head" in the sense of being imaginary. They are very real. The presence of symptoms may, of course, mean that there are unidentified, hidden physical abnormalities. These are not discoverable because medical science has no tools and tests to do so. And even if they are discovered by some future test, that doesn't necessarily mean relief. Therefore, the pursuit of discovering these potential, yet unproven, abnormalities cannot be a patient's main goal.

I mentioned at least two reasons for the inability to find discernible tissue abnormalities and damage (see chapters 2 and 3): the body is not flawless and medical science and scientists are limited in its and their ability to discover the cause of symptoms. There is nothing perfect in life, including a person's body and medical science. There will always be more symptoms than discovered causes. Therefore, try as they might, doctors are just not able to find the cause of every symptom in the body. So when I use the term "nothing wrong in the body," I mean that nothing was found or discovered in the body that was thought to be the reason for the symptoms. Most often the symptoms are attributed to emotions out of control. When that happens the person's thinking and wanting are not considered important as to the origin and persistence of symptoms.

There is another reason why symptoms may be present when nothing is found or discovered wrong with the body. The symptoms of "feeling bad" and pain may also be produced by how he uses his body in responding to various situations in life. They are produced as a result of his thinking and attitude about the present situation. This could include his thinking as he laments that medical science is limited!

For example, a person may have a headache. As a response to perceived or actual pressure at work such as a demanding schedule or boss, he tenses and tightens his muscles in the head and neck. This use of the muscles and physical response of his body produces symptoms. However, at other times, even though he is not at work, he may have the same pain. This time it comes from the unpleasantness at work (pressure) that constantly nags at him even away from the office. This same pain also may occur without tense muscles.

Consider another example: the athlete or performer is about to go on the field or stage. Prior to his performance, he experiences pain and cramps in his abdomen. This was a regular occurrence with me before my high school football games! I was always told that these were "butterflies" and that I would be okay after the game got going. As I reflect back on those times, I know now that I was thinking and wanting certain things. I was concerned, even worried and fearful about my performance and the results. I focused on the outcome and possible failure. This type of thinking and wanting has its focus on control and is termed "stage-fright," worry, and fear. The way I was thinking and the content of that thinking affected how my body felt and the symptoms I experienced.

It is instructive to look at what happens when anyone has pain and focuses on the discomfort and restrictions of his activity. Recall from chapter 2 that there are connections in the brain between the center that receives and sends pain signals and the *attitude or thinking center*.[a] This helps explain why what a person thinks affects not only how he feels, but also how he feels and senses pain. So often, people call this emotional pain. If anything, feelings are running rampant because thoughts and desires are focused on something that the person has not gotten and may not get. Again the issues are one of control and resources. If you focus on how unpleasant and miserable you are, the severity of the pain only increases (this was discussed in chapters 2 and 3; see footnote, page 22).

Likewise, many people who limit their activity because it "hurts" find this approach to pain relief unhelpful. Limiting physical activity is often accompanied by increased cognitive activity. Thoughts are focused on the badness of the situation and limitations that often are self-imposed. The net result is an aggravation of the pain complaints.

---

a   There is not one pain center in the brain. Rather, multiple areas of the brain, including the thalamus, frontal cortex, and limbic system, are involved in the recognition, evaluation, and interpretation of the pain impulse. Initially, the thalamus receives and sends messages to other parts of the brain, specifically the limbic system and frontal cortex, the latter being the *thinking* or *attitude* center of the brain. The limbic system is composed of various parts of the brain (amygdala, hippocampus, septal area, and cingulate cortex). This system is involved in the processing of cognitive and emotional information and its expression.

In a similar manner, the thalamus is connected not only to the *attitude center* but also the *emotional* or *feeling center* via the limbic system. This helps explain why a person's feelings affect his response to feeling pain. If a person is upset (such as sinful anger, sinful far, and worry which is always sinful) for any reason (such as pain hindering his ability to do what he wants), this may also aggravate pain.

In summary, in this life no one can escape pain, but his response to it (which is what he can control) will greatly influence its intensity.

It is also helpful to look at what happens to thinking when there is or there is thought to be no known relief for pain and no known cure for the condition causing pain. As he thinks about and reflects on his situation, all he can see is a future of pain, more pain, loss of ability to do what he would like to do, and no potential relief. In short, he longs to return to his previous state. He wants what he may not be able to get. He measures success by removal from his "I don't like" situation. The situation is not the issue. The issue is his response. One reason given is to regain function. Some patients express it this way: "I want my old body back." "I want to be young again."

Based on the fact that "my old body and my previous function are gone and may never come back," a person may conclude that things are hopeless. He then feels sad, grieved, upset, and frustrated, thus producing more bad feelings including pain. And when he considers other life problems, it is easy to become even more hopeless. The end result of this downward spiral is depression, which in turn only aggravates the pain. Making any effort to deal with the condition seems useless. Depression is a feeling state marked by a certain type of thinking and wanting. It is produced when people focus on unpleasantness of their situation and conclude there is no hope. In response they continue to let their feeling be their guide. They give in to feelings and give up on responsibilities and others. Bad feelings are the reasons given for this activity or inactivity. Actually they give up on God. They picture the mountain so high, the hole so deep, and the tunnel so long that no end that desire is in sight. As believers, they live the lie (Psalm 42-43; John 14:1-3).

So depression is really the result of how one has handled many difficult aspects of life. The person has looked over his situation and made a judgment. That judgment was based on his hopes, wants, expectations, fears and goals. He then came to a conclusion: "My situation is hopeless." The person uses his selfgenerated hopelessness and feelings to determine thoughts, desires, and actions. I the end, depression has no proper vertical reference. The reasons given are the feelings and God's providence – the person's situation.

Now that the person acts as though life is hopeless, all that is left is "somehow to go on with life as it is," "get by," "tolerate it," "do the best I can," "keep looking for relief," or "try to squeeze a little happiness out of a miserable life." He may even quit functioning and take to the couch for a "pity party." He has given in to his feelings. Depression, then, is not only giving up but giving in to how one feels.

All of this can be true especially when one has a disease that includes any one of the rheumatic disorders. A person's outlook may stem from failure to experience the relief he wants in spite of treatment. In response he expresses his thoughts and desires in various ways including resentment, bitterness, anger, and fear. He may focus on such things as no cure, uncertainty re: his family, and cost. It is easy for him to become discouraged. Continuing this negative focus which is a focus away from God toward self makes it easy to give in to the feeling of hopelessness, which we have said is depression.

A difficulty I face as a physician as I listen to and care for patients is summarized by these comments: "I don't think myself into pain." "What does attitude have to do with it anyway? It's my body that is the problem. Just fix my body and I'll be okay." "I am a good tolerator of pain. But this pain is just too much."

This line of reasoning is based on a number of misconceptions. One is that "nothing is wrong in the body" means that the symptoms are imagined, not real. If this is true, then I would be calling the patient a liar. I have made the point, here and elsewhere, that only a person himself knows if he has pain or not. Symptoms may or may not be accompanied by demonstrable abnormalities. However, neither of these facts means that the patient is not experiencing what he says he is experiencing. I help people understand the concepts of something wrong in and with the body.

Another misconception is the belief that a person is only body. When someone tells me that attitude is not important or that he is not thinking himself into hurting, I ask him to tell me how he concluded that. The answers are varied but generally center on the idea that: "I don't have any problems in life." "I don't have marital problems and things are okay at work." "I tolerate pain well and I don't go around making myself hurt."

The response that he has no problems in life or in his marriage indicates the belief that wrong thinking occurs only in response to "the big things" in life. Rather, it is one's response to everyday situations, events, and people that are sometimes termed pressures and strains of life that help expose wrong attitudes and thinking. And everyone has pressures and strains. These range from bodily problems and pain, to cars that won't start and next door neighbors that may not be the friendliest.

So I ask the patient: "Are you just body? How are you different from an animal?" The patient often tells me, "I try to get my mind off the pain by doing something different." After I ask that question, then I pose another: "What have you learned about thinking, wanting, and pain?" The patient then begins to make the connection.

I often hear from patients: "I tolerate pain well." I ask them what they mean by that and hear something like this: "I have always been able to handle pain but this is different: it is longer and harder." And because the pain is perceived in this way, the assumption is that there must be something wrong in the body. And therefore: "My attitude and thinking don't affect my pain."

Based on the statement that the patient tolerates pain well, I ask her why she is here. "This pain is different – more intense and more threatening." She is telling me that she handles, or more accurately, responds to certain things including pain differently. I ask: "What is different about this pain than some other pain?" That question takes us back to the influence of a person's thinking and wanting and their influence on hopes, expectations, and goals.

The above mentioned patient has perceived her particular pain as "terrible" and "worse" because the pain and her body are considered liabilities. Achieving her hopes, expectations, and goals is hindered. Her conclusion is that life is frightening and hopeless.

Another response I hear from patients is this: "The pain depresses me. I wasn't depressed until the pain came." I then ask: "How did the pain do that?" Their response reflects their underlying concern:

"I am not able to function as I want." Maintaining function, as the patient defines it, has become his main goal in life. It is as if a pain-free or pain-limited existence this side of heaven is a right for the person but for Jesus Christ. Anything that threatens this is perceived as bad. This is where the *boomerang effect* shows up (see chapter 3). It is caused by thinking about the pain that precedes the increased intensity of the pain when pain relief and a return to *normal* function are not forthcoming.

Most medical people teach that depression is the result of something wrong with the body. However, a physician makes the diagnosis of depression simply by listening to a person's description of how he feels and by observing his behavior. There is no clinical or laboratory test to prove there is something wrong with the body. Physicians often say depression is due to a "chemical imbalance," or a brain problem based on some neuroimaging study report. The basis for these statements is based on theory and mostly conjecture given such a strong desire to follow the Medical Model. This model is based on finding some anatomical or physiological which can explain not simply symptoms but explains the an underlying pathology. There is no laboratory test to verify the supposed imbalance. In addition, no one has explained what this imbalance is. Is it too much? Is it too little? What is out of balance? How many of what chemicals are out of balance? What does it mean to be out of balance?

And even if a chemical imbalance should be found, there is no proof that the chemical imbalance caused the person to think or act or even feel the way he describes. No studies have demonstrated consistent changes and if any changes are the chicken or the egg in terms of the cause or the effect of bad feelings, in fact, the possible imbalance may be the result of the bad feelings rather than its cause. Since depression cannot be measured, like blood pressure or blood sugar or weight, there is no proof that a chemical imbalance exists or caused the feelings that are used to diagnose depression. It may seem logical that there is a chemical imbalance, or neuroimaging abnormalities, but it is not necessarily good science nor is it helpful..

Now a word about *stress*. What is stress? The term can be tricky. Medical science speaks of stress and a stress response[19] and tends to consider them the same. Those influenced by psychological thinking define stress as "any event that strains or exceeds an individual's ability to cope."[20] Those influenced by this sort of medical thinking state:

> The concept of stress is now well accepted within the scientific establishment. It can be quantified more accurately using a variety of tests. Stress is a complex, dynamic situation in which normal homeostasis of the internal milieu is disturbed or threatened. This disturbed state can be induced by a variety of intrinsic or environmental stress triggers which may be psychological or physical (e.g., pathogens, toxins) and to which the organism must respond to maintain physiologic equilibrium.[22]

This author is stating to us that stress is something that occurs in the body in response to the threat of unpleasant circumstances. Consider a person that is injured in a car accident. Arriving on the scene, the paramedics find that he has multiple injuries. As a result, there will be things happening in the body in order to protect bodily function and keep it as close to normal as possible. These changes can be measured and occur no matter what the inciting stimulus. The same physiological response occurs when the threat is pneumonia or even a heart attack.

It is in that light that such medical science also speaks of a *stress response* as what goes on inside the body especially in regard to two systems: one has to do with higher brain centers (hypothalamus-pituitary-adrenal axis) and the release of hormones, and the other with the autonomic nervous system (see footnote, page 22). Each system functions to maintain a homeostasis in the body that is desirable and preferable in order to continue the normal balance of the body. This is usually termed *adaptation responses*.[a][21]

What does all that mean? How should we understand it? Simply this: certain chemical changes occur in the body as the person reacts to any number of situations considered unpleasant or threatening (medical and psychological science call them *stress* or *stressors*. I call them *pressures* and *God's providence*). These chemicals, such as cortisol, have various functions, can be measured, and are part of the physiological stress response.

However, cultural teaching would have us believe that something outside of the person (the situation itself) makes him respond and feel a certain way. This teaching theorizes that the individual is not responsible for his thinking, desires, actions, and feelings. Those things just are as part of "normal" physiology. Stressors, then, relate to external circumstances that the individual must think about, process, and then draw a conclusion. Pain and bodily problems are included in the category of stressors.[24] Medical theory doesn't attempt to explain the connection between particular feelings, including pain, and stressors, except by way of physiological changes that occur in the body.

---

a   "Regardless of the source of stress, the body mobilizes its defenses to ward off the threat in a pattern referred to by Hans Selye as *the general adaptation syndrome*." Lahey, p. 504.

However, when patients who visit my office speak of stress, they are referring to something going on inside of them that they are confronting. The fact that they are responding to pressures however defined is remote to their thinking. Even more remote is pressure is actually God's providence. They are aware of at least two things: pressures around them (which they call stress) and uncomfortable and unpleasant symptoms (which they may also call stress or stress-related). They connect the two by cause and effect. They speak of being under stress. They are willing to attribute, and even blame, their symptoms on stress.

The person has assumed, wrongly, but in agreement with medical theory, that "stress also causes you to do things that intensify your pain, such as tense your muscles, grit your teeth and stiffen your shoulders. In short, pain causes stress and stress intensifies pain."[25]

If this is true, then a person is at the beck and call of things outside of him. And if that is true, where is hope? It can only be in changing that which is outside. How hope-generating is that? Very little, because changing others and situations is usually impossible, and the resulting victim mentality only leads to bondage.

It is true that responses to pain, in terms of thinking, wanting, doing, and feeling, can be accompanied by measurable changes in the body. However, it doesn't follow that pain causes a certain way of thinking or even certain feelings. A painful condition may make it easy for a person to think and desire in a certain way but it is not causative.

Patients who think this way have wrongly attributed power to that which is outside of themselves. They have lost sight of the connection between how they feel and their desires, thoughts, and actions. Moreover, God's providence comes in all shapes and sizes. A response to them is a response to God. They have failed to understand, and perhaps accept, that symptoms do occur as a result of their reactions to little things in life as well as big ones.[a]

I have also heard this from patients: "I am not under any stress except this pain that is always there." Patients who speak this way emphasize what "my pain has done to me and not allowed me to do." They then say, "It takes a real effort for me to do. I try to accept it – that I have pain and can't function like I want." Patients who speak this way have failed to understand that bodily problems and changes in the body's functioning require a response on their part. These people, too, have failed to understand the connection between wanting, thinking, acting, and feeling.

Consider another person who was "under stress." He described various trials and tribulation, other terms for God's providence. He described that which was outside of him and his response. This person is the Apostle Paul (2 Corinthians 4:7–10; 6:4–10; 11:23–28). It is clear that Paul's circumstances were difficult. These included physical threats and harm to his body, rejection by his own people, and times of an uncertain outcome for him and his friends. From his perspective there was much uncertainty in his life. He knew the final outcome but not the steps leading to that outcome.

How did he respond to this pressure? I suspect physiological changes were happening in his body. I suspect chemical neurotransmitters and

---

a   The term *accept* and *coping* are used quite commonly today. What do they mean? Usually patients explain it this way: "I have pain and a body I don't want but, I must get on with life." These terms don't spring from a person steeped in biblical hope and they are not hope-engendering themselves. In fact, the only hope is getting rid of "this bodily problem," which may not be possible. A patient explains how he tries to cope – he accepts it: "I ignore my pain," "I get busy," "I try to take my mind off of the pain." In other words, coping is applied accepting. This means "sucking it up," "grinning and bearing it," and simply existing until he gets rid of this bodily problem. The hope is change and the change is defined as pain relief. Patients who use these terms don't understand biblical hope as Paul did.

his brain scan would show activity. The same surmise could be made regarding Jesus Christ. But no matter. Those things were not important or God, in His Word, would have made it clear to us. What is important is the Holy Spirit's teaching on this subject of pressure. Paul was not a victim of his circumstances.

Paul believed God's promises. He had a choice: to act on those promises or, in effect, depress himself. How? He could choose to focus on his pain: his difficulties and hard times. This would lead to despair, hopelessness and depression, which is failure to function. I had a patient who said, "I don't need anything to depress me. I can depress myself about anything in life." Rather, Paul joyful chose to believe the Scriptures and trust and obey in spite of feelings by fulfilling his ministry responsibilities. What motivated him to make this choice? He responded this way out a growing love and knowledge of God and out of of gratitude for God's grace to him (2 Corinthians 4:1).

Therefore, I must dig deeper to discover what is going on with a patient: What is the patient thinking, wanting, fearing, and hoping? So I ask: "What do you mean by the word *stress*? How do you define it? How is it unpleasant?"

The most common answer is that the person is experiencing some unpleasantness or an "I don't like" situation. Once I understand that, I pose this question: "What is it about that particular pressure and unpleasant situation that produces new or increased pain?" Invariably, the person's thinking and wanting takes center stage. What he desires drives his thinking, which then influences his feelings (including pain) and his actions. Things external to a person can influence how a person feels in his body because of his desires and thinking.

However, there is no credible evidence that things outside a person make a person think and feel a certain way. Make, determine, and influence are not synonymous. Therefore, it is correct to talk about pressure (look at Paul's case) as that which is outside of a person to which the person responds. That response does affect the body and how a person feels and behaves. Based on my definition of stress (pressure from the outside AND a person's response) an unbiblical response to pressure or perceived pressure is what causes a person to feel stressed. Physiological changes may be demonstrated in the body. The statement: "I feel pressure or pressured" describes the person's thinking or attitude to what I call an "I don't like" situation. In fact, describing it as an "I don't like" situation means he is already thinking a certain way.

His thinking and attitude are influenced by his desires and wants rather than the outside pressure. The outside pressure is the context in which his desires and wants are expressed. In chapter 3, I made the point in reference to thinking and wanting and pain perception by using three illustrations – a bear, a call from an IRS agent, and a secretary at her desk. If the person *chooses* to respond based on unbiblical wanting and thinking, then the results will be an unbiblical reaction that will affect the body. These bodily changes that can actually be measured include heart rate, skin temperature, and intestinal activity as well as elevated levels of certain chemicals such as cortisol.[23]

To repeat then, stress is a person's unbiblical response to pressure being that which is outside a person. Physiological changes occur and can be felt by the person and can be measured (such as a fast heart rate). Actually, the whole person, inner and outer man, is responding.. This unbiblical response does affect the body and some of these changes may be felt by the person. Pressures involve those situations in which the person's control and resources for responding are the issues. Some examples of pressure include: unfulfilled desires and wants that may have morphed into demands; unmet expectations; and goals or success points that are in danger of being fulfilled.

A word here regarding responses and reactions to various pressures. While all responses have a cognitive component (thinking element), some indicate a greater degree of reflection than others. Sometimes reactions are immediate and almost second nature – the patient says, "I was not thinking." Of course that is incorrect. All people have mental activity. However, there is value in distinguishing between immediate and long-term responses to pressures and the unpleasantness one experiences. Responses can and do change and that simple fact is a source of hope, especially for patients trapped in the web of seemingly unending pain. The key is change: but change into what?

A person may not be able to do much to change his body in terms of the disease or condition, but there is much he can do to help change his response. What hope is available for a person in dealing with his reality? The wisdom of our culture has its own way of viewing pain and bodily problems and of determining hopes, fears, wants, expectations, and goals; it claims that this view offers much hope. What is the contemporary view of pain and bodily problems? What wisdom does it attempt to bring to the hurting person? Is it really what it claims to be? Answers to those questions will be the subject of the next chapter.

CHAPTER FIVE

CONTEMPORARY WISDOM AND CULTURAL ANSWERS FOR THE PROBLEM OF PAIN

WHEN ANYONE IS FACED WITH the daily task of living with and in a body he does not like, he is looking for help. There are many sources offering their brand of help. What happens when someone like you is faced with the reality of having pain, in a body he doesn't like, which will remain with him for the rest of his life? Often, he will turn to the contemporary wisdom of our culture for help and answers.

For that reason alone, it is important to see what the wisdom of the culture has to offer. Another reason to look at this subject concerns the results of acting on those answers. So we must ask ourselves: Where do the culture's answers lead? Does the person achieve his goal of pain relief? And if so, at what cost? But perhaps the greatest reason to explore this topic centers on the goal of the culture's wisdom regarding pain and pain relief. Is the goal of pain relief an inferior goal even if there is pain relief? How would one determine the answer to that question? Is there a superior goal that is obtainable even when pain relief doesn't come?

So what are the answers of our culture? What are the results of seeking these answers? The answers and help offered are dependent on the view of pain and the one offering help. The assessment of the problem yields the solutions offered. In other words, how contemporary society views a certain fact determines what help it will offer. It is no different for pain.

What is the contemporary cultural view of pain and bodily problems? In general, our culture's assessment is quite simple: pain is bad and it has no useful purpose. Therefore, when chronic pain is present, the focus must be on removing it. It exists to be stopped. The adage is, "Do your best to get rid of pain; don't let it control you but you control it." The emphasis is on you for the purpose of removing something considered undesirable.[26] So often self takes center stage.

In addition, we are advised, "Get what you want: Lead an active, and productive, more normal or better quality life you deserve." That is only done through pain relief, which is accomplished by a person taking charge of his life. The culture encourages him to seek help in doing so. Where is that help found? It is found in any number of places including the doctor's office, the psychologist's office, group therapy, distraction, imagery, visualization, meditation, self-hypnosis, cognitive behavioral therapy, physical therapy, medications, pain clinics, self-help books, the Internet including social media, and inpatient hospitalizations.

One book reports that "No longer is pain viewed as just a symptom of another disease. It can become an illness in itself."[27] Another publication states "Chronic pain is not a meaningful signal. There is no injury. Chronic pain is garbage in the brain."[28] Still another publication reports the following:

> Pain is a problem of enormous magnitude in the United States. According to a 1996 Lewis Harris Report, 46% of all Americans experience severe pain at some time in their lives.

For these Americans, pain has a profoundly negative effect on quality of life and psychosocial well-being. Notably, research has shown that pain does not necessarily need to be intense or severe to produce significant decrements in quality of life; even mild or moderate pain may have a detrimental effect. Pain not only diminishes psychosocial well-being, it reduces functional capacity as well.[29]

No wonder that pain is public enemy number 1. So, I ask again: "What is society's view of pain and how does it play out in our culture?" A plethora of medications, self-help books, inpatient pain units, and pain treatment clinics highlights society's approach to pain: it is to be understood, removed, conquered, and overcome.

Although there are a number of current approaches to pain relief, I have found that they share common features. These include:

1. The patient is labeled a chronic pain sufferer.[a][30]

2. There is an emphasis on the personal nature of pain.

3. There is an emphasis on the fact that pain always affects the chronic pain sufferer's life in a negative way and that the effects of having pain are always bad.

4. Therefore, pain relief and returning the person to a normal, active, productive, better quality of life in spite of pain is the goal. (However, normal, productive, and better quality of life are not defined except in terms of pain relief).

Society and the medical community takes a multifactored approach to pain relief. This includes a patient's commitment of starting to take control of pain; beginning a program of either inpatient or outpatient

---

a   In fact, patients can be labeled as chronic sufferers depending on the organ system involved. This is done using a diagnostic code number from the International Classification of Disease coding manual. This allows for reimbursement.

treatment; dealing with *emotions* and thinking of the person as he views life, pain, and his bodily problems; managing *life stresses*; and fitting people and things into a schedule and strategy aimed at getting pain relief and a better quality of life for the person. There is an emphasis upon "the power within to motivate you to a better, higher comfort zone of pain relief."[31] In addition, there is an emphasis on the use of medications, administered by various routes, to give the person what he seeks and thinks he deserves to make him feel better with a better quality of life.

With this multifaceted approach to pain management, the message given is: somebody has heard the patient, somebody cares, and hope is available if the person so desires. It is also clear that pain is bad, has no useful purpose, and exists to be removed. If pain can't be eliminated from the outside using medications, injections, and possibly surgery, then a person has inner resources available to do his best to get rid of the pain. If the pain remains, then control of it is the goal so it will not control him.

Basically, medical science approaches pain by concentrating on pain relief and considers what is the best method to give the person what he wants. The authors of self-help books, either from personal experience or from caring for patients who complain of pain, realize that typical approaches such as medications, injections, and surgery are not effective in giving pain relief.

In other words, people still complain of pain. The figures in chapter 1 support that fact. One author writes: "Frequently, though, none of these approaches is effective. The pain lingers, despite repeated trips to doctors and various efforts to stop it. However that doesn't mean there isn't any hope."[32] The hope presented by the author is a "hope so" hope. And it is given in terms of pain management. His goals for people who report persistent pain are to manage the pain and improve their quality of life. The term *quality of life* is usually defined in terms of pain relief and, sometimes, more function with less pain. Doing something about the pain takes center stage, so that there will be less complaints about pain.

To that end, and in an effort to be helpful in giving "hope so" hope, other ways to reach those goals are reported. These include educating the patient about the body's pain system and body mechanics, and stressing the role of attitude and lifestyle. Basically, the thrust is to accentuate the positives and minimize, if not avoid, the negatives. The positives in this case are: for the person in his "inner self" to be attuned to managing his emotions, asserting himself, and giving himself the proper self-worth and esteem.

In almost any material on the subject of chronic pain, a chapter concerning "taking control of your pain" will be included. "But it is up to you to make it happen (living active and productive lives) . . . You are the key ingredient."[33] The emphasis is on you, to take control of your pain and it is your choice. Again, self takes center stage.

Research and the practical experience of caring for patients who have persistent pain indicate that education is important to promote understanding, compliance, and patient satisfaction.[34] Such education typically teaches the anatomy of pain pathways and transmission, pain perception, the physical effects upon the body of limited physical activity (bodily deconditioning), and the value of certain types of exercise.

Education is also directed at recognizing the costs of chronic pain, sometimes described in terms of the *rippling effects of chronic pain*. [35] The cost of chronic pain is categorized as physical deconditioning, loss of sleep, emotional upheaval, depression, difficulties at work, financial strain, damaged relationships, and chemical dependency. The emphasis is on what pain has done to the person and what he "can do to help minimize these personal and economic costs and, in some cases, avoid them."[36]

The importance of attitude and thinking is stressed. The connection between the inner man and the outer man is acknowledged. But not in biblical terms. Achieving the right balance between thinking and doing is urged in order to have the best quality of life and minimize the pain. Techniques of mind control include imagery, visual inner healing, distraction, meditation, and even spirituality. All are endorsed as acceptable alternatives for facilitating pain relief. The idea goes something like this: "Since pain is a matter of personal perception, only our mind knows what pain and comfort is. Imagination is the access into your subconscious mind. Your imagination is not something that is simply there but is a kind of hidden energy. So use it."[37]

What are the results and success rates of these types of treatment based on contemporary wisdom? Varying success rates for improvement of pain and pain relief can be found in different sources. However, the words "chronic" and "persistent" indicate that people continue to face pain that motivates them to continue to seek help. Pain and its relief continue to be focal points in this present society.

So why may people report improvement in their pain levels and feeling better using these approaches to pain and pain relief? First, medications do affect the the body and often in a variety of ways. For example, narcotics or opioids block pain receptor in the brain and spinal cord. However they also block the body's own ability to produce endorphins. As a result, patients often report less pain relief and the medication is increased. It is thought that medications reduce the feeling and sensation of pain through these and other mechanisms. So subjectively and symptomatically, people can feel less pain and, therefore, report improvement. Second, the human being is a unit: mind and body. He is not one or the other. Therefore, what he thinks affects pain perception (see chapter 2). Most attribute this phenomena to "the power of positive thinking," "mind over matter," or the placebo effect. God's creative design is not acknowledged and these terms flow from poor anthropology and function as a Creator-denying method of pain relief.

As God's creature and image-bearer, man was designed to function as a unit. The "mind over matter" philosophy means that thinking both in the inner and outer man exerts control so that what goes on in the body is ignored or denied. The person actively and cognitively engages both his thinking, wanting, and doing with the goal of reducing his awareness of pain. Please remember that man was designed as a duplex being – inner and outer man. Man is a unit. Therefore he has a body but he is not body. He has a spirit or soul but he is not only spiritual. The Bible teaches that man thinks, desires and acts as a whole person — in both his inner and outer man. Therefore thinking and wanting are linked to feeling including pain and vice versa. We correctly say that the Bible teaches that it is not "mind over matter" but God's word through the Holy Spirit in union with Christ that leads to proper thoughts and desires.

I understand that human beings do what they do and feel what they feel because they think what they think and want what they want. This makes sense because the Bible, not human "wisdom," tells us that man is a unit, body and spirit, and functions as such. Experience has simply borne out this biblical truth, but this unit must be controlled by God's Word, not by "positive thinking." The terms positive and negative thinking generally to their effect on pain and pain relief. However, those terms could not exist unless God designed man as a whole person, inner and outer man.

Third, the result of "mind over matter" is a self-focus. When self and self-satisfaction take center stage (as these methods and approaches to pain relief suggest they should), then attention and thinking is diverted away from the pain.

Fourth, this self-focus motivates a person to keep looking for what he really wants and thinks he needs to be happy: that is, pain relief.

Fifth, there is a victim mentality that accompanies the label "chronic pain sufferer." These people are caught in the web of an "I don't like" situation and they are doing the best they can to extricate themselves. It also appears that the concept of victimhood appeals to some people.

Consider once more the following statements: "I can't function because of pain." "I just want this to go away so I can get on with my life." "I don't have time for this." "I have so many things to do but can't get them done." "Stress makes my pain worse." "Pain makes me nervous and depressed." "I am a good tolerator of pain and doing the best I can." "I don't want to depend on medications." "If this much pain is present now, what is going to happen in the future?" Stop and ask yourself: "Is this all there is to life?" "What if I can't get pain relief?" "Is there anything better?"

Now consider the results of seeking pain relief as the major goal in life. In the middle of pain, all too often the desire for pain relief is all-consuming. As a result, the pain manages, even controls, the person.

Think of the mornings. Many a patient has told me, in so many words, that the course of his day is set by the presence or absence of pain when he awakens. If he has no pain, he sets off on daily activities, wondering when pain will come. If there is pain, he makes plans to deal with it, handle it, cope, or just get by. A cycle has been produced that dominates and controls his day. What is the result of all this?

First, there is constant awareness and pondering: "How much pain relief and for how long?" There may be minutes, hours, or even days of little or no pain. However, when the wondering sets in, this only heightens concentration on pain, and pain appears or gets worse. This may create the desire for more pain relief. That result is exactly the opposite of what the person is trying to accomplish, and pain returns or worsens. This is the boomerang effect (see chapter 3, page 37). A focus on pain, as we have seen, generates more pain (see chapter 2, page 22).

Second, since medications are being used, there are always questions: "Will they work?" "For how long?" "When will I need another pain pill, and what will be the result?" There may be side effects from the taking of the medications, anywhere from a slimmer pocket book (cost) to effects on the body. There may be a dislike of taking medications, especially for something that the person doesn't like and doesn't want. All of this only heightens the awareness of pain as the person concentrates on eliminating it. This lifestyle is futile and, in the end, unsuccessful.

Third, what about other people associated with the pain sufferer? The person who has pain may well view other people through the eyes of his condition and pain. Consequently, they will be used as helpers to get by or hindrances as they may get in the way of pain relief. Again self takes center stage and relationships are affected and often strained.

Fourth, visiting physician after physician is a common occurrence: "Just one more MD who may tell me what I want and need to hear and give me some hope in finally getting pain relief." This desire for pain relief holds the person in a grip that enslaves. It is insatiable. A little bit of pain relief is never enough.

The picture is not a pretty one. Do you see and understand the endless, hopeless futility of the pursuit for relief that promises much but provides little? The net result that I hear from patient after patient is one of frustration and discouragement. Those who desire pain relief and set out to gain it, pursuing what the culture promises, usually don't find it. Patients believe and even convince themselves that a little relief is better than none, and live their lives as if all that matters is just a pinch of pain relief. This is bondage.

I ask again: "Is there anything better? Is it even possible to live life not controlled by pain or the pursuit of pain relief?" Everything within, and much around us, says that pain relief, even though not permanent and only short-lived, is what a person should seek. Why is that? Because basically, people are convinced that they would be happier and could accomplish more if they hurt less. Thus, it seems reasonable to pursue pain relief. However, as mentioned in earlier paragraphs, that approach is futile and counterproductive in the end. It simply does not work. The result of the desire for pain relief and the pursuit of that desire is a cycle of want, demand, need, expectation, disappointment, and more pain. This cycle only aggravates the situation. Even if relief comes, the course of a person's life may be so etched in the suffocating straight jacket that more is better or at least the status quo must be maintained.

An emphasis on pain relief colors a person's thinking as it leads to a self-pleasing desire and vice versa. That is displeasing to God and repulsive to others. What each person needs is something to help him determine what is best. What he needs is direction outside of himself; he needs biblical guidance and counsel.

Before we leave this topic, let me add a closing note so I will not be misinterpreted. The issue is not whether seeking pain relief and using various modalities to achieve it is legitimate or not. The key thought is taking care of the body in order to please God and to serve one another. Seeking pain relief is not necessarily wrong (see chapter 3). Good stewardship of the whole person often includes going to the doctor. Seeking pain relief as a good steward is always godly.

To the preceding, I add this: some of the approaches presented under my discussion of the contemporary view of pain and pain relief may even be reasonable and appropriate (the discussion of which ones and how used is a topic for another time). As with any desire, the rightness or wrongness of the desire for pain relief can be evaluated by looking at what happens when you don't get it, or by what you are willing to do to get it. When you don't get what you want, how do you respond? Why do you seek pain relief and what methods are you willing to use?

It is when the various methods and maneuvers for getting pain relief become fundamental to decision-making that they are wrong. Generally, this occurs in people labeled as chronic pain sufferers whose pain relief has become a major motivating factor in their lives. However, this same desire can occur in people whose pain is considered acute.

So what is better than pain relief? Is there anything that is like a breath of cool, fresh air in the midst of a hot, humid summer day? Is there anything that offers hope and help in the thick of things? Is there anything that provides answers for a life that seems complex and unanswerable? This subject will be discussed in chapters 8 and following. But first, the next two chapters will address the subject of spirituality and pain. So buckle your seat belts tightly and hang on. What is in store for you is "oh so simple" and yet extremely profound.

CHAPTER SIX

SPIRITUALITY AND PAIN PART I: DEFINING SPIRITUALITY

THE PURSUIT OF PAIN RELIEF leads people down many different paths. One of those paths is the use of complementary and alternative therapies (CAM). Spirituality, which I define later, is considered one of these CAM. I suspect you, or someone you know, have been tempted to investigate or try one of the many CAM.

Still, you may ask: "Why is it important to discuss this subject, especially in a book addressing the topic of pain?" The answer to that question is twofold:

1. The Bible defines spirituality and gives it direction to its significance. Because this is the case, you must use a biblical grid to sift and filter what the culture teaches. Otherwise, what man thinks, in contrast to God's wisdom, becomes authoritative. Before accepting the conclusions of contemporary wisdom, we must define what that wisdom is. It is no different when considering spirituality, healing, health, and comfort.

2. Secular writings agree that spirituality is important. In fact, society is busily writing and talking about it. Therefore, many believe that spirituality has a place in the care of patients, including pain relief. However, biblical spiritually is not the focus

of this agreement. Rather, spirituality as defined by the culture competes with spirituality as defined by the Bible.

Some professionals are recommending spirituality (however defined) for comfort, health, and healing. Both nonmedical and medical communities believe that spirituality has an effect on the body. I concur; spirituality *is* important, not only in the area of pain, but for *all* of life.

In this chapter, we will consider the "pro" side and take up the culture's call to "use" spirituality to get healing, comfort and health. After summarizing various sources addressing this topic, I shall conclude the chapter with seven biblical truths, including a definition of spirituality. I will then draw three conclusions based on those truths. In the next chapter, I shall consider the "con" side expressed as concerns and even objections to the use of spirituality for the purposes of healing, comfort, and health.

These CAM are generally considered unconventional and unproven, at least by the bulk of the medical community. These therapies are multiple and may vary depending on the disease and condition being treated. Interest in CAM has exploded recently and continues to escalate.. The reasons are many and include:

1. The increased frequency of chronic and incurable diseases and conditions in all age groups as well as the growth of an older population;

2. The failure of conventional therapies to defeat death, disability and suffering, and the side effects that accompany such conventional therapies;

3. The yearning by patients for effective, simple, safe treatment options;

4. The desire of patients for pain relief and the control of their destinies in the face of an uncertain future regarding their conditions; and;

5. The desire by patients for therapies and practitioners that are "natural" and holistic[a] (see page 80);

6. The desire of financial gain by producers.

One author writes:

> So compelling are these issues that the overwhelming majority of Americans with chronic diseases will, at some time, try complementary or alternative therapies or practices regardless of their disease, education, background, or socioeconomic status. The prevalence of complementary and alternative practitioners and widespread use of these practices cogently reflect on the current limitations of our science and our art.[38]

The goal of any therapy is to improve the patient's situation and condition. All therapies must meet some test or tests of validity. Most practitioners, but not all who promote various therapies, use scientific methods to confirm this validity. The call by the medical community is that therapy be "scientifically grounded and evidence-based."[39] However, those who promote CAM rely on subjective statements of improvement recorded by those taking the treatment.

But questions surface when the reported "improvement" of a patient's condition is defined. When the goal is pain relief, or relief from any symptom for that matter (such as fatigue), then this subjectivity becomes the final authority by which to judge benefits. Attempts to

---

a   I don't favor the use of this term as its users are trying to indicate man is a mixture of many parts. Rather, the Bible views man as a unit – inner man and outer man – not divided.

measure how one feels by any objective standard are unsuccessful and even futile. There are no pain gauges, fatigue meters, or joy thermometers. No matter how hard a person tries to objectify symptoms, the end result is still subjectivity as a standard if not *the* standard for judging benefit and improvement.

Terms for such benefit such as *quality of life, feeling better, doing better,* and the vehicle for getting there, such as *coping, coping strategies,* and *acceptance,* begin to take on an air of sophistication. If these goals are reached, the therapy is considered successful. Pragmatism (using that which does "work," however defined) then assumes a far more significant role in the care of patients. The question: How do you objectify the subjective? The answer: You don't; and you can't no matter how you try.

So why do medical people continue to try? One answer would be the desire to give people what they think they should have and want, for whatever reason or reasons. Another answer emerges from the mindset that every symptom means a bodily defect that can be and deserves to be corrected.

So given these thoughts, what should one think about CAM? One physician states it this way:

> Despite concerns about the perceptions and credibility of
> these practices, several increasingly compelling reasons are
> evolving. Our patients have made it clear that they are interested in CAM. These individuals need care and guidance, and
> the alternatives they seek need assessment. To ignore this
> is not fair to our patients and is imprudent for responsible
> physicians. The challenge is no longer "Should we think
> about this?" but rather, how do we do so in a manner that is

objective, credible, and sensitive to the needs of our patients and professional communities.[40]

The remainder of this chapter and chapter 7 addresses the validity of this statement.

To begin, let me repeat what I said in the opening paragraph. It is important for us to investigate this subject given the orientation of society and the medical community toward pain relief, subjectivity, and pragmatism. Because "everybody is trying it," it is important to stop and see just what the culture's spirituality is and place it against God's standard, the Bible.

Health professionals are aware that the outcome of any disease may be dependent on factors other than the disease process. Consider the patient who is confronted with pain and a body he does not like. Fear, anger, and frustration are common responses but they are not universal. Patients are often said to be "in denial," "failing to cope adequately," or "not accepting their condition." But not every patient responds the same way to any particular disease. If the condition or disease is the same for each patient, then how does one explain the different responses?

It is interesting that most health care professionals recognize that a spiritual dimension exists for each person. A common term for this is *spirituality*. The fact that man is spiritual is in accord with the biblical teaching that man is not simply material (body) but inner man (spirit) as well. Yet most of these professionals do not further acknowledge that this truth results from the essential nature of man as created by God.

The culture's definition of spirituality is God-denying or at least God-minimizing. The Bible teaches that man at his very core was created a spiritual being. He is body but not only body. He is spirit but not only spirit. Rather, he is a duplexity: a unit consisting of both body (or material) and spirit (or inner man). In the Bible, the inner man is referred to by a variety of terms including mind, will, affections, spirit, and soul. Man's inner man is where he thinks, hopes, fears (as well as other emotions), purposes, doubts, considers, and decides on courses of action. Moreover, man is a worshipper. He worships himself through the affection for and devotion to some object, thing, or person.

A common term encountered in the medical literature that attempts to include the truth that man is a spiritual being is *biopsychosocial*. It emphasizes the fundamental importance of psychological, environmental, and spiritual factors as determinants of health.[41] However, this concept doesn't acknowledge the full biblical teaching of man's spiritual nature, and ultimately leads to an unbiblical compartmentalization in understanding the patient and in caring for him: the doctor deals with bodily issues, the psychologist with psychological ones, the social worker with societal ones, and so on.

The term does, however, point out that man is more than body; he is a person – immaterial spirit plus material body. Some would call this view *holistic*. Indeed, the Bible tells us that man is a unit and functions as such. What a person wants and thinks influences what he does and how he feels. Said another way, a person does what he does and feels what he feels because he thinks what he thinks and, most often, he thinks what he thinks because he wants what he wants.

Biblically speaking, man's desires, thoughts, and choices originate in his heart, the inner man. Only later does his brain, an organ of his body, transmit corresponding signals to the rest of his body. Therefore, efforts to produce appropriate behavior by changing a man's brain and its activity (such as with drugs or surgery) are doomed to failure. Such a designation is a another attempt to bypass God's design of man.

Man's moral compass isn't located in the brain, but in the inner man – the heart – which the Holy Spirit supernaturally changes so that man thinks God's thoughts, desires what pleases God, and acts accordingly.

I mentioned that physicians and health care professionals are aware that factors other than the disease itself are important in patient responses and the outcome of their disease and condition. These variables are termed *psychological, emotional,* and *social* factors. They refer to inner-man issues (the heart) including thoughts, desires, and intentions. The origin of inner-man issues is not in the brain and the body. There is no word for brain in the Bible, Old or New Testaments. The brain is part of the outer man. When considering these issues, you begin inside and work outside – from the heat and to body including the brain. Unless you do, the patient and physician will "confuse: God's solution with those given by and through contemporary wisdom.

The terms *psychological* and *emotional* carry much baggage in today's world and should not be identified with anything biblical. We must begin with the Bible, its study of man, and God's solution for troubled people in a troubled world. *Social* factors are, in reality, the context in which inner man's concerns intersect and collide with the situations and circumstances of life. Social factors are actually God's providence. They are the context in which a person demonstrates a desire to apply God's truth in order to please God. These concerns come to the surface when the person is faced with trouble and include wants oftentimes masquerading as "needs." What a person wants or does not want is exposed in the heat of daily pressures of life. Bodily problems are part of the heat coming at people.

A one-line summary up to this point would be this: the culture teaches that since man is a spiritual being, spirituality and the quest for it may influence pain, disability, and bodily problems. In fact, according to this definition of spirituality, a spiritual approach to health and disease is quite common in today's society.

The success of 12-Step programs such as Alcoholics Anonymous, which rely heavily on a 'spiritual' approach, provide direct evidence of the potential value of spiritual approaches to medical conditions. A review of the medical literature, particularly the family practice literature, suggests an increasing interest in exploring the relationship between patients' spiritual needs and more traditional aspects of medical care.[a][42]

Having determined that the issue of spirituality is prominent in society and in the medical community, how does one apply it to the area of pain and pain relief? The first issue is the term *spirituality*. What is it, how does one define it, and where does one go to do so? Once a person's source for understanding spirituality is pinpointed

---

a   I comment on the 12-Step movement by quoting from two sources, William Playfair in: *The Useful Lie*. Crossways Publishers. Wheaton. 1991. p. 86, and Martin and Deidre Bobgan in: *12 Steps to Destruction*. Eastgate Publishers. Santa Barbara. 1991. p. 71. First, from Doctor Playfair: "Many within the Christian community believe that the founders of AA were Christians and that AA's Twelve Steps are based on the Bible. The 'Higher Power – 'God as you understand him' – referred to in the Twelve Steps is, according to this myth, none other than the Most High and only God of Biblical revelation. However, nothing in AA's history supports these beliefs. In fact, the myth is actually denied by the founders themselves as well as the official literature of AA and spin-off organizations." And second from the Bobgans: "The first Twelve-Step program was devised by Bill Wilson. Alcoholics Anonymous began in 1935, when Wilson and Dr. Bob Smith invented a road to sobriety. Three years later Wilson began work on a manuscript that would become known as the 'Big Book' of Alcoholics Anonymous. Until the publication of the book, most of what was done in AA was by the word of mouth. In codifying the system for the book, Wilson divided the general principles of AA into Twelve Steps. "Wilson originally wrote Twelve Steps for alcoholics (a convenient euphemism for drunks), but eventually others adopted and adapted the Steps in an effort to overcome their own addictions (a convenient euphemism for lusts and habituation). Later the Twelve Steps were applied to all those who lived with or worked with people with such addictions (life-dominating sins). Thousands of groups across America use Wilson's Twelve Steps and most codependency/recovery programs utilize Twelve Steps in one way or another." While AA and spin-off groups are dependent on faith, thus making them religious (even spiritual), this spirituality runs counter to our biblically derived definition.

and spirituality is defined, then the questions to ask are: Is a spiritual approach to medical conditions just one of many approaches that a person can use? Is a spiritual approach one that may serve man admirably if it works but which should be put back on the shelf if it does not? Is it something that can and should be used even, and especially, if the desired results of pain relief does not occur? Is a spiritual approach the same thing as applying biblical principles to all of life? If not, then what is it?

Another question to ask before jumping into the arena of a spiritual approach is: Should one take the plunge? If the answer is "yes," then what will a person do with the information gained in his investigation? To answer these questions, one need only survey the numerous articles both in the lay press and medical press addressing spirituality, religion, disease and health. Not only are articles being written and printed but national conferences on the spiritual aspects of health are common. Therefore, one can assume that the issues of spirituality, religion, disease, and health are part of the mindset of using all possible avenues to get relief from pain. We must jump in to discover what authors are saying about the subject.

Spirituality has been defined in different ways. No definition uses the Bible as the authority and source for its definition. Often spirituality is taken to be synonymous with *religion*. However, most articles cite a difference, and define *religion* as: "any specific system of belief, worship, conduct, etc., often involving a code of ethics and a philosophy."[43] This is then distinguished from spirituality.

On the other hand, "spirituality has to do with man's search for a sense of meaning and purpose in life; it is that part of a person's psyche that strives for transcendental values, meaning and experience."[44]

"While spirituality often flourishes within religion, this association does not alter the independent nature of each concept."[45] This author goes on to say: "Spirituality may be found in a personal relationship with God which goes beyond the social processes of religiosity."[46]

Spirituality is also defined in existential terms, as the experience of interaction with individuals, society, nature, the universe, or spiritual entities. In addition spirituality is represented by "the pursuit of an ideal."[47] The author previously quoted concludes that there are common themes in the definition of spirituality that include: "relationships (for example, with others, God, the universe), an interconnectedness, a meaning in life, and a strong belief/principle system. Spirituality is a concept that acknowledges that there is a real finiteness of self, but that accommodates the uniqueness of self."[48]

Another author attempts to simplify matters by stating: "The spiritual dimension is that part of a person that allows God-consciousness and the possibility of relatedness to God, however God may be defined."[49] "Spirituality can, therefore, be portrayed as a conscious or unconscious belief that relates the individual to the world and gives meaningfulness and definition to existence."[50]

"Pain practitioners are beginning to focus attention on the complex interrelationships between health and treatment outcome."[51] Why? The same author speaks very clearly when he says: "Successful pain management programs teach how to eliminate unnecessary pain and suffering, allowing them to cope adequately with residual dysfunction and loss. The ability to cope is affected by many psychosocial factors including underlying neuroses, self-image, acceptance and fulfillment of the role expectations of society, family interactions, the meaning one attributes to the experience comprising life and the quality and depth of one's spiritual foundation."[52]

The overarching goal and purpose of many pain practitioners is to use spirituality and/or religion to bring about health, healing, or comfort: to make a person feel better, even good. We will see where that goal takes us as we look at what other authors say.

"Polls indicate that the U.S. population is highly religious; most people believe in heaven and hell, the healing power of prayer, and the capacity of faith to aid in the recovery from disease. The popular press has published many articles in which religious faith and practice have been said to promote comfort, healing or both."[53]

The question might be asked: Why not use religious activities, especially if they work? This is the "what's in it for me?" approach to the "Christian" life and it is followed by both medical and non-medical people, believers and unbelievers. Help is defined as better feelings. Do only medical persons model this approach? Unfortunately, many churches apply this approach to both the churched and unchurched. Too often, the call the call is to come to receive Christ because of what "He can do for you." People are pressed into worship services because of what it will accomplish for them. Anyone can then ask: If churches today approach worship, service, and evangelism this way, why not use God for my health, comfort, and healing?

R. P. Sloan and his co-authors, commenting on the upsurge of interest in the effect of the spiritual dimension of man in the lay and medical press and the subsequent recommendations of various authors, cite " . . . three stated or implied justifications for making religious activities adjunctive medical treatments: religious activity is associated with good or improved health; such activities provide comfort and patients want their medical care to include attention to religious matters."[54] The goal of their article was to: "demonstrate that attempts by physicians to integrate religious interests into medical practice are not nearly as well justified or simple as the literature suggests."[55]

More will be said about these comments in the next chapter as we hear Sloan and his colleagues represent the "con" side of mixing spirituality and medicine. For our purpose now, their comments serve to stimulate thinking critically on this subject.

These writers first address the issue of "empirical evidence of a link between religion and health."[56] They point out that the strongest evidence of an effect of religion on health comes from studies using church attendance as evidence of religiosity. Their concern focuses on the definitions of spiritual and religion: "Religious services are diverse in style and content as the difference between a Quaker meeting and a Roman Catholic mass illustrates. Do advocates of the connection between religion and health propose that such differences are unimportant?"[57]

The same questions can be raised regarding faith and prayer of Christians, Jews, Muslims, and others. Sloan and his co-authors close their article as follows: "Most important, we are concerned that attempts to obtain scientific evidence of the health benefits of religious activities and to use such activity instrumentally in achieving beneficial health outcomes not only are superficial but also suggest that the value of religion derives from its effects on health. Religion is more important than a collection of views and practices and its value cannot be determined instrumentally; it is a spiritual way of being in the world."[58]

Post and colleagues defined spirituality as *faith in a higher being* and pointed to Gallup polls to highlight the resurgence of spirituality in the United States. They cited two reasons for addressing what he called faith-spirituality in the treatment of patients: (1) "When patients feel that their spiritual needs are neglected, . . . " they will seek other care; (2) certain subspecialties of medical science have " . . . established that such emotions as anxiety and hope can be factors in illness outcome. The keys to emotional coping with serious illness and disability are frequently found within the matrix of patient spirituality."[59]

Post quotes an Islamic study indicating the benefit of " . . . spirituality in its religious form." A Muslim physician regarding patient requests for prayer, and a rabbi wrote: "Disease forges an especially close link between God and man; the Divine Presence Itself, as it were, rests on the head of the sickbed."[60]

An article published in *The Annals of Internal Medicine* addresses the matter of religion and medicine under the format of a "contemporary clinical issue."[61] The author reviews information from various writers who have written and spoken on this subject. The subjects covered were faith and healing, prayer and spirituality, the "if" and "why" debate first debate and discussion on the measurement of the effects of religion and spirituality, the search for an explanation of "why" regarding the link between religion/spirituality and health, and the medical community's response.

The author's bottom line is recorded in the last paragraph of the article: "Whatever their position on these issues, most people would agree that a physician's own beliefs are important. That is, physicians must be comfortable with the idea of introducing religion into the practice of medicine before they take any further steps. They should not feel pressured to do anything that conflicts with their deepest beliefs."[62]

Sloan and colleagues believe that religion should have an extremely limited role in the physician's office.[63] But note, however, even these authors acknowledge some role! They reach this conclusion because of the "very poor empirical support" that exists. Sloan and colleagues disagree with other authors who claim empirical support for "improved health" using various spiritual maneuvers.

In addition, they express concern that "religion in the office" "raises all of these ethical issues."[64] In other words, "using religion or spirituality" (however defined) in the office borders (if not being outright unethical) on the unethical (however defined). He and his co-authors are also concerned with "trivializing religion," which is "Treating religion like another medical intervention." They say: "Religion does not need science to justify its existence or appeal";[65] "Prayer is seen as a relationship with the Almighty"; and "To engage in that relationship for what a person can get out of it, namely health, is a misuse of that relationship."[66]

These authors have concluded that physicians are not trained (qualified?) to correctly bring God and religion to bear on the patient's medical condition. Again, more will be said in the next chapter regarding these comments and conclusions. However for now, juxtapose the statement "very poor empirical support" with "religion does not need science to justify its existence or appeal." While it may seem admirable that some people do not want to treat religion as another medical intervention, they are using medicine's rationale of pragmatism: "Does it work as determined by experience and empirical, scientific data." This, in effect, is regarding medicine as another religion.

What is one to think and do having reviewed some of the available material? The crux of the issue is really simple (not simplistic): Where is one to turn for direction and guidance for life regarding the issue of spirituality and religion? We have addressed that specifically in this chapter and also throughout the book. The answer is: To find guidance for life, turn to the owner's manual called the Bible. Or as Isaiah said in Isaiah 8:20: "to the law and to the testimony!"

A major focus and emphasis of the Bible is a proper definition of spirituality and its influence on people. As I have said, man is a duplex being, body and soul or spirit. The Bible directs the believer into a proper understanding of spirituality. The Bible addresses the issue of pain as part of God's control and judgment and a proper response to it. The Bible is about spirituality, and the Bible is about pain and "I don't like" situations. Therefore, let us set out several Biblical truths:

1. All of life is theological, as man was created to receive guidance and direction from an outside Source, specifically, God Himself. Adam, in a perfect world, with a right relationship to God, and no sin, was given guidance and direction about life.

2. This God is the one, true, living God who has revealed Himself in His Word, the Bible.

3. God is the God of the Bible and not just as some person claims to know Him. Rather, God knows Himself and has recorded what He says about Himself in His Word, the Bible.

4. Man is a religious being and a worshipper. How could he not be, if God is his Creator and man is the image of God? Thus, God has something to say and that something is binding and authoritative for all men everywhere.

5. Spirituality must be defined by using God's truth found in the Bible. Anything else is a poor, feeble substitute. Therefore, when

religion is defined as worship of anything other than the God of the Bible, it is not biblical spirituality.

6. Biblical spirituality means being indwelt by the Holy Spirit. This indwelling occurs after He has implanted the principle of new life (regeneration) so that the person now becomes a believer. That means he is a new creature in Christ (2 Corinthians 5:17) and in relationship to Christ. This relationship is personal and intimate.

7. The believer is led by the Holy Spirit (Galatians 5:16–18; Romans 8:14) to do what the Scripture prescribes. Being led means a change occurs in thinking and behavior. The Spirit enables the believer to resist the desires of the "old man" (old lifestyle) so that the deeds of the flesh are not produced.[a] Rather, the fruit of the Spirit is more and more evident in the believer's life.

Based on these simple yet profound truths, one should conclude that it is intellectually (and spiritually!) dishonest to say that it is wrong to bring religion into any area of life including the practice of medicine. In fact, the statement, "no religion in the office," is itself a religious statement. It purports neutrality and attempts to protect religion. The statement reminds one of Albert Ellis and his "shoulds and oughts."[67] Ellis advocated that there should be "no shoulds or oughts" and yet what he does is espouse what he would prohibit. "No religion in the office" is similar to the U.S. public school system as currently defined by the federal government and the Supreme Court. Under the guise of neutrality, religious freedom, and tolerance, the U.S. public school system has imported its own religion.

---

a   The old man is the old person – the old person that you were in Adam before conversion. The old man includes the old lifestyle: thinking, wanting and acting. Some may refer to the old man as the natural man.

A second conclusion would be that one should not be against religion in the doctor's office: it is not possible for the reasons given above. The central issues then are: What religion? What spirituality? What does it look like? What form does it take? How does a doctor present it to the patient? What follows in the next several chapters attempts to spell out answers to each of those questions. My source in answering these questions will be God's owner's manual – the Bible.

A third conclusion is that man is a whole person, both inner man (heart, mind, spirit, soul) and outer man (body) and functions as such. Religion, to be helpful, must address both outer and inner man and base what it says on truths given to us from the Creator of both. The Bible clearly teaches who God is and does not leave this open to vote by individuals or committees. God is the central focus of all life. Pain and bodily problems come from His hand, for His glory and the believer's good, and everyone must give an account to Him on Judgment Day. As we shall see, those truths make all the difference in the world to the believer experiencing pain. His relationship to God, not some nebulous higher being, impacts his daily life as he uses biblical principles to respond to both hard and good times.

CHAPTER SEVEN

SPIRITUALITY AND PAIN PART II: APPLYING SPIRITUALITY

WHAT ARE THE WAYS TO help get pain relief? Patients, their families, and health care professionals often turn to any approach that "works." The discussion in chapter 6 focused on the specific contemporary and alternative therapy of spirituality. There are those who view spirituality/religion as effective and even good medicine, enabling a person to achieve comfort and pain relief. I opened the chapter with two major reasons for considering this subject in a book concerning pain. I concluded the chapter with seven biblical truths and gave three conclusions based on those truths.

From the start, and it cannot be repeated frequently enough everyone has a belief about God, self, others, and life. Everyone is in relationship to God whether acknowledged or not. Man is a spiritual and physical being (he is a duplex being). Therefore everyone is a theologian and life is theological, always with a vertical reference whether acknowledged or not. The Bible is the only authoritative, accurate, and trustworthy definer of proper theology meaning and significance of spirituality. As I described towards the end of chapter 6, spirituality means being indwelt by the Holy Spirit (Romans 5:5; 8:9-13). There is the implanting of a new orientation, direction, and disposition of life (called regeneration, new birth, new life, quickening or awakening; see John 3:3-8, Ephesians 2:4–6).

As a result, the whole person becomes a new creation and a new existence in Christ (2 Corinthians 5:17). This means he has a new orientation, tendency, inclination, and bent with the capacity to please God rather than self. He is so influenced by the indwelling Spirit that the believer turns from the deeds of the flesh and self-serving and self-pleasing (Galatians 5:16–25) to serve the one, true, living God and bear the fruit of the Spirit.

As was pointed out in the preceding chapter, the various sources referenced do not use the Bible in defining spirituality. Therefore, all conclusions drawn from those sources about spirituality and its effects on health are limited and inaccurate. Those sources are the result of human reasoning and thinking, the view of medical science, and the interpretation of what society thinks. The reason to discuss the topic is not because the medical and secular world are doing it, nor even that positive results have been described using spirituality. Rather, the purpose in discussing spirituality and medicine is to do justice and honor biblical truth and the God of that truth concerning spirituality, stewardship of the whole person, and God's answers to the effects of the curse of sin in this world.Therefore, any attempt to bring help and hope to hurting people must originate in and be interpreted by biblical truth.

Later, I will return to the issues raised by Sloan and colleagues previously discussed. I will use their voices as representing the "con" side of spirituality and medicine, including the "use of spirituality in the office," as a platform for presenting further biblical truth. In addition, I intend to use the concern of Sloan and his colleagues for the proper use of one's relationship to God as a springboard for discussing certain lines of thinking presented in Christian writings. From that point on in the book, I will focus on what the Bible has to say about spirituality, health, comfort, healing, and pain relief.

Some writers on the subject are concerned with "going beyond" religious bounds. The concern of trivializing religion or spirituality was raised by Sloan and colleagues. How did that concern arise? (1) Sloan reported that spirituality is more than religion, (2) the effect of religion/spirituality on health cannot be measured using empirical, scientific methods, and (3) using a relationship to get something such as health or healing was a misuse of the relationship.[68] Let's look at those three concerns in closer detail.

Certainly, one can see that spirituality (whether biblically defined or not) and religion (outward expression of one's spirituality) are not the same thing. The secular literature makes that point.[69] The greatest reason for beginning with the Bible is to honor God and His creational design which gives the most benefit to the person. What does God say about spirituality is the most fundamental question any could ask. In emphasizing this point Jesus brought the Old Testament teaching to center stage (1 Samuel 15:22–23; Isaiah 1:10–17; Hosea 6:6–7; Amos 5:21–24; Micah 6:6–8). Jesus condemned those who attempted to separate the condition of a person's heart (inner man's condition from external activity; Matthew 9:13; 12:7; 23:1–32). Jesus pointed to true spirituality which changes the whole person. Jesus taught that true spirituality is Holy Spirit wrought and energized (John 3:3–8; 6:60-64).

What does this mean? Here is where one must define his source of truth or his epistemology. So ask yourself: "From where do I draw my conclusions about life?" That choice, in and of itself, is a religious and theological endeavor. Everyone brings to those choices certain presuppositions and beliefs. These are functional belief systems based on a standard of truth.

Cornelius Van Til, a Christian apologist, successfully argued that everyone thinks, reasons, and argues circularly, with his presuppositions as the starting point and frame of reference.[70] One will always return to those initial presuppositions. A mindset emerges with certain thoughts that impact one's interpretation and problems, including pain and bodily problems. Consider Hebrews 11:6:

> *And without faith it is impossible to please God, because any-*
> *one who comes to Him must believe that He exists and that He*
> *rewards those who earnestly seek Him.*

The faith the author speaks of in Hebrews is saving faith, which is a gift (Ephesians 2:8–9) and has God as its object. Saving faith is a a gift mediated by amazing saving grace whereby an individual receives and rests upon Christ alone for salvation. Saving grace is never alone. It is associated with the fruit of the Holy Spirit and sanctifying grace. There is life after salvation. Both saving and sanctifying grace is manifested by the person's response to God's truth about the good news which is found in His Word, the Bible.

Man was made a believing and trusting being so that all human beings have faith: they believe and trust. The issue, then, is not whether one has faith but what the object of that faith is and how it is exercised. Both religion and spirituality are based on faith because man is a a faith-based being.

Saving faith is key for any discussion of spirituality. Spirituality can be properly defined only by the believer (because he alone has received the gift of saving faith). Therefore, for the believer, spirituality must be defined by using biblical truth. Anything else is a substitute and a poor, feeble imitation.

What about measuring the effects of religion/spirituality using empirical scientific methods? Is it possible to measure the supernatural by the natural? Some authors have said, "yes," but Sloan and coworkers say, "no." Sloan and colleagues seem to be referring to a supernatural or even miraculous effect on the body, either directly or via thinking. However, it depends on a person's definition of supernatural. In my use of the term supernatural, I include God's work in the inner man. It is possible to tell who regenerated people, changed from the inside out, are because they think, desire, and act differently. In fact, according to 2 Peter 3:18, there must be tangible evidence of growth.

The relation between the observable or external and the internal was a source of confusion for the disciples. Consider two occasions. One is recorded in John 4:31 through 34 (more will be said about these verses in chapter 9). In these verses, Jesus had concluded His conversation with the woman at the well. The disciples returned as she was leaving. They encouraged Jesus to eat so that He might be satisfied. They were quite familiar with the enjoyment of physical satisfaction, the pleasure of eating, and the subsequent feeling after a good meal. Jesus threw them a curve ball.

How so? Jesus introduced them to the concept of suprasensual satisfaction (v. 34) rather than sensual satisfaction. Simply, Jesus said that pleasing His Father was a far superior satisfaction and delight than what they experienced when they finished a good meal. He encouraged them to think and "see" with the eyes of faith, (suprasensually), rather than by the senses (sensually). Paul gives a brief commentary on Jesus' teaching in 2 Corinthians 5:7. The believer walks by saving faith –

spiritual eyes illumined by the Holy Spirit – and not the physical eyes. Jesus was a good steward of His body. He was not against eating. He was for something far superior, the wonderful satisfaction of pleasing His Father by trusting and obeying Him.

A second example is recorded in the first three books of the New Testament (the Synoptic Gospels). The gospel writers recorded Jesus' interaction with the rich young man (Matthew 19:16–30; Mark 10:17–30; Luke 18:18–30). The issue was salvation. The young man wanted to know what he had to do to enter heaven. Jesus gave a simple answer: perfect, perpetual lawkeeping. Jesus recited that part of the Ten Commandments that addressed doing and not doing. The young man was still not satisfied. In fact, he reported that he was an excellent law-keeper even since childhood.

So what now? To this point, the disciples had been tracking with Jesus, observing the give and take of the conversation. In fact, they understood exactly where the young man was coming from. The facts (that could be gathered by the senses) were there for all to see. The facts, as they understood them, coincided a the works-based religion (Galatians 3:1-3; Philippians 3:3-6). But then Jesus dropped a command that pierced to the young's man heart. It dealt with the suprasensual. He told the young man to divest himself of anything that hindered his allegiance to the one, true, living God. This command penetrated not only to the very core of the young man's being, but to those of the disciples, as well.

After hearing Jesus' words, the young man left deeply distressed. Jesus turned to His disciples and said, "It is hard for a rich man to enter the kingdom of heaven" (Matthew 19:23). The disciples did not understand. They asked: "Who then can be saved?" Jesus explained: "With man this is impossible but with God all things are possible." Jesus was teaching that the source of truth is outside of a person. Submission to this source of truth was far superior to anything the disciples could sense (with their senses), and the result of this submission brings satisfaction and contentment not only in this world (salvation), but also in the future one (Matthew 19:28–29; 1 Timothy 4:7–8).

So what about applying scientific methods to determine whether religion and/or spirituality "works"? Should one do it? Can one do it? And why would one want to do it in the first place? First, one must define "works." Second, he would have to agree that works should be the standard for effectiveness. And third, one would have to ask: What does the Word of God say about health? What are the results of good stewardship of the body?

The Bible teaches that God is for the body (1 Corinthians 6:13ff).The believer's body is a temple of the Holy Spirit (1 Corinthians 6:19), that he is to present his body to God as an act of logical service (Romans 12:1–2), and that his body is not his but God's Who expects a return on what He has given (1 Corinthians 6:20; Matthew 25:14–30; Luke 19:11–27). Therefore, he should do all for the glory of God (1 Corinthians 10:31). Elsewhere the Bible teaches that the best thing a believer can do to promote good health is to function as a good steward by applying such principles that are contained in passages such as Proverbs 3:5–8; 15:30; 16:24; 17:22.

Viewing Jesus hanging on the cross, broken body and all, might in-dicate that God made a mistake – that He is not for the body or that a believer's body should never suffer as Jesus' did. Some are even bold enough to ask: "Did God make a mistake in allowing Jesus to have His bodily problem?" "Did He fail Jesus?" Closer to home, you might ask: "Did God make a mistake allowing me to have the body I have?"

Man's logic is no match for God's. One's understanding of the cross comes only from the Holy Spirit's applying His Word to a changed inner person so that the person begins to think God's thoughts after Him. Then one realizes that God's purpose and intention in the cross was not to reverse the curse of sin on the body in this life (2 Corinthians 4:16–18). The reversal of sin's curse on the body is a blessing to be received in future glory, and the way to that glory is through the cross (Romans 8:18; 1 Peter 1:6–9; 2:19–21).

Rather, bodily problems come precisely because God does not now choose to reverse the curse of sin. In fact, it is the believer's calling (1 Peter 2:19–21) and privilege (Philippians 1:29) to suffer for Christ's sake. It is God's purpose to have the believer use hard times and trouble as His instrument for the believer to grow (Romans 5:1–5; 8:28–29; James 1:2–4; 1 Peter 1:6–8) and to honor Him in other ways.

So, the Christian should go to the doctor, not primarily to get well or for pain relief, but to be a good steward of the body (chapter 5) – this pleases God. Preventing illness, getting well, and pain relief may be by-products of one's stewardship of his body. Learning and applying what the Bible teaches about good health is good stewardship. The simple truth is that a right relationship to God in Christ does more to promote good health than anything else.

Yet, even this does not guarantee that a person will be free (or healed) of bodily problems. As the cross demonstrates, experiencing bodily problems with all the pain and uncertainties that accompany these problems, is God's road to glory: His and the believer's (see footnote page 102). If God designed the body and is the Creator of the body, then what He says about the body has to be just what you need to know about it.

From our review, various sources imply and even encourage using spirituality as an alternative or adjunctive approach to bodily problems for healing, comfort, and health. The movement and thrust of the marriage between religion and/or spirituality and medicine have focused on the results, and those results have focused on getting: healing, comfort, and health.

When the Bible's definition of spirituality is used, the issue focuses using the Bible's definition of spirituality then, the question focuses on the believer's relationship to God: Is it to get or receive something or is it to give honor and glory to the God of the Bible? What is the value of a relationship with Christ through the Holy Spirit in this life and the next? The issue is not whether the believer receives anything in return on this earth. In fact, he receives much – but it is not necessarily healing and comfort (1 Timothy 4:7–8). The issue is where does one begin to evaluate whether a relationship with God (or for that matter any other person) work?

So, what is the purpose of the believer's relationship with God? How you answer this question depends on your view of God and what you think you need and want in this life and your eternal destiny. The question itself poses difficulty. Would you bring the question to Christ as He hung on the cross? Would you pose that question to the Father as darkness filled the land?

Sloan and his colleagues, I think, correctly raise the issue of the purpose of relationships. However, this is not new. God Himself raised it. The Old Testament message is stated clearly in Isaiah (42:8; 48:9–11) and in the first and second Commandments (Exodus 20:4–6; Deuteronomy 5:7–10). God will not be used. He is no cosmic dispensing machine, nor a robot or bell boy to enter a person's service at his beck and call.

Rather, God has a plan and agenda. God the Father sent His Son, the incarnate Christ. He came as the unwelcome God reclaiming what was rightfully His (the believer's very heart) as the great Rescuer saving a people for Himself to and for His own glory (Philippians 2:6–11). His people share in His glory as they share in His suffering (Philippians 1:29, Romans 8:18). Why? Because every believer is united to Christ since God established a relationship between the believer and Christ.

So, when Paul says in Romans 8:17, that believers are children and heirs, he also speaks of believers as fellow sufferers (which is the road to glory). The Greek word for suffering is *sumpascho*, a compound word with its root, *pascho*. This word means "to be affected or afflicted by something from the outside" or "to be acted upon" or "to have an experience."[a]

By definition, every believer has had or will have an experience similar to that of Jesus Christ by virtue of his relationship and union with Him. In another sense, every believer (but also every unbeliever)

---

a A word is in order regarding the road to glory. Paul speaks of believers as fellow sufferers with Christ. The Greek word, *pascho*, means "to suffer." It is the word used for the suffering and death of Jesus (Luke 17:25; 22:15; 24:26, 46: 1 Peter 2:21; 3:18; 4:1). Then, is suffering the only road to glory? If the answer is "no," you will be tempted to grumble and complain when you have problems with your body that don't go away. If the answer is "yes," you may be tempted to exalt suffering and the sufferer. So how are we to understand that answer? By understanding suffering. Suffering is a result and consequence of Adam's sin. It is part of the curse. It may result from a believer's own sin. Unbelievers also experience suffering as the universal result of the curse of sin. The road to glory for Jesus was the cross. There was no other way. After His life and death, He arose, ascended, and then He returned to His rightful position at the right hand of the Father. Jesus' own words indicated the absolute necessity for Jesus to suffer and die (Matthew 16:21; 17:23; 20:17–19). Consider believers. Is suffering the only road to glory for them? In one sense, yes. How so? The believer is in Christ (see chapters 8, 9, 10). That means union with Christ. What Christ did, the believer did. What Christ experienced, the believer experienced. What Christ accomplished, the believer accomplished. Secondly, God has not reversed the curse of sin even for the believer. Thirdly, an attack on the believer and the church, for Christ's sake, is an attack on Christ (Acts 9:4–5; 22:7–8; 26:14–15; 1 Corinthians 12:27; Ephesians 1:22–23). However, we must not equate our suffering with Christ's. A believer will never suffer separation from God. A believer may never experience Paul's thorn or Job's physical afflictions. And, it is not necessary to do so. What is necessary is to submit and obey, applying biblical principles even if it costs pain. A proper understanding of suffering is given in Acts 5:40–41. The disciples rejoiced in their suffering because they were considered worthy to be dishonored on behalf of Christ. Joy was the result of knowing that they could suffer in honor of Christ.

will experience pain and suffering as part of living in a fallen world with a sin-cursed body. The believer can experience hard times and pain as Christ did. Since the believer is united with Christ, he can think, evaluate, and respond in a way that honors God and is Christlike – he grows and changes. This change is known as progressive sanctification – being gradually set apart from sin and self to God. God will not treat His children any differently than he did his Son in terms of trouble. Constantly Jesus was faced with the choice of pleasing self or pleasing the Father. The believer will not bear the cross of God's wrath as Christ did. The believer is to put to death self-pleasing as Jesus did. Since the cross is an instrument of death, the believer will die to self as he bears the cross of self-denial. He denies himself that which he wants – to please himself. As he grows in Christlikeness, he will find more satisfaction in pleasing God that in pleasing himself. More on that in the following chapters.

God had an eternal purpose in sending Jesus: to save a people for Himself for all eternity. This eternal purpose impacts the life of believers daily, orienting them to hear, understand, and respond to such commands as Paul gives in Colossians 3:1-3:

> *Since, then, you have been raised with Christ, set your hearts*
> *on the things above, where Christ is seated at the right hand of*
> *God. Set your minds on things above, not on earthly things. For*
> *you died, and your life is now hidden with Christ in God.* (see
> also Matthew 6:33; Romans 6:11–13; 8:18).

The "things above" are God Himself and the eternal inheritance He is keeping for His people (1 Peter 1:3–5). The prospect of seeing God face to face in eternal fellowship. The daily life of the one who sets his heart on heavenly things is presently motivated by a future certainty. It is only then that he is of earthly good.

Scripture teaches that the believer's relationship with God was established by God and exists primarily for His glory (Ephesians 1:3–4, 9–10; Revelation 4:11). This fact returns us to the original question posed by Sloan and colleagues: "What is the purpose for one's relationship with God?" Let me be clear that we are talking about a believer and His relationship with Christ. Let's listen in on my conversation with a patient in the office on a routine day.

—You are telling me about your pain. What have you done in response?

—I have talked to God about it.

—Tell me about that.

—I prayed and still pray to Him. Without God and my faith, I would not be able to cope. He helps me tolerate the pain and get by.

—What do you pray for?

—For relief and to get through the day.

—What has been God's response?

—Well, I still hurt.

—So what do you think His response is?

—Well, I guess, no. But I keep praying.

The patient usually understands that God's answer has been "no." However, most have not thought through His "no" and their response to that "no."

Here is an opportunity to apply the biblical principles found in 2 Corinthians 12:7-10. There, Paul, acknowledged God's sovereign power in causing (or allowing) his physical problem. He knew its source (v. 7). He also acknowledged that God's purpose was for his good – to prevent him from sinning (v. 7). Paul did pray earnestly for healing. He knew God heard and answered every prayer – yes, no, and wait. Praying for pain relief and healing is not necessarily unbiblical. However, what was Paul's response to God's "no"? He looked beyond the pain to the gain, which was to experience God's help and grace in a way he could not when he was physically well. Therefore, Paul got excited – not about his physical problem – but about the opportunity to grow and change. His response to God's kind explanation is nothing but supernatural. In response and because Paul understood God's plan for him and all believers, Paul prayed trouble. What in the world was going on? Paul knew that trouble was the crucible for his growth in Christ. He desire for growth in Christ was greater than his desire for relief. Relief came as he focused on pleasing God.

When a person's focus is concentrated on the desire for pain relief and the hope and desire that God will give it to him, he will focus on the pain rather than the gain. So in my conversation with the patient, I ask:

—What has been your response to His answer?

— When pain relief doesn't come, I take a pill, usually a nerve pill or pain medicine, and do the best I can.

What is the patient saying? Basically, he is saying: "All I want out of life is a little help now and then. What is wrong if I take a pill to relieve me?" In response, I ask:

— What are you saying about your relationship with Christ?

That is a bottom line question. It cuts to the heart and soul of the person sitting across from me. On reflection, most will attempt to retract the statement and may present the same thought in a different manner. For example, a person will say something like this: "I didn't mean that my pill was the same as my relationship with Jesus Christ. What I mean is that I just need a little help every now and then."

How are you to interpret the "help now and then" approach – especially when God has said "no"? Is it wrong to take medications when you are hurting? To answer those questions, we must go to God's Word. Consider Paul's response in 2 Corinthians 12. What motivated Paul? Was it an "unmet need" or his desire to please God? Knowing that he and every believer was re-created to please God helped him view himself and the circumstances through God and His purpose and not vice versa. It was to know God, please Him, and live for Him (2 Corinthians 5:9, 14–15; Philippians 3:7–11). Based on that motivation, Paul gloried in God's "no." He saw a good God and His purpose and knew that purpose was for his good. Therefore, he could and did glory in God's "no" to him.

The desire to eliminate pain is like any other want that has been elevated to a place of status and authority for a person. With that mindset and *functional want system*, a person will use whatever means is available to get what he wants and thinks he must have. The means for getting it can include God Himself. God, then, serves as a tool to be used and worshipped for personal gain (God becomes an idol).

One such mindset is the victim mindset accompanied by certain needs. The idea is that circumstances "do it to me." The person's supposed "needs" (which are really wants and what he thinks he can't do without) come in all shapes and sizes. And one can put a pious twist to this by looking to God to satisfy them.

Another view holds that every believer has a redemptive right for good health and that it is a matter of a person's faith (Matthew 8:17). This right was received at salvation. The curse of sin on the body is alleged to be removed in this life. If that fact does not materialize the person must generate more faith but what that looks like is never defined. If one believes that healing is a right, then one will pursue obtaining that right by whatever means he can find – even using God to get it. Pain will always be seen as an enemy, never a blessing. The cross will be seen as something remote and impersonal. Often the means of getting healing is by attempting to generate faith on top of faith. He will try to persuade God to give him the healing he claims is his redemptive right. Obtaining this right controls the person.

When healing does not come because God has said "no," the person may not want to take "no" for an answer. The issues here are how you respond to God's "no" and why. There is biblical precedent for persistence in prayer (Luke 18:1–8). Going to God in prayer can be a demonstration of your dependence and confidence in God. But your response to His answer is also a demonstration of your trust and confidence in His wisdom, power, and purpose. The desire to be free of pain should not be separated from a desire to please God by being a good steward of the body. When that happens, the desire becomes inordinate by focusing on what you want. If that is the case, you will respond in any number of ways. You will expend an increased effort to generate more faith (as if God needed your faith to bring about healing). Or you may grow weary and hopeless, thinking God has let you down. This can lead to the downward spiral of thinking discussed in chapter 4. The result is hopelessness, apathy, increasing frustration, pity parties, and usually more pain. Or you may become angry and bitter. You may say the anger is not at God but at the problem. In truth, you are angry at God. A response and reaction of anger always carries with it the mindset that: "It is okay for me to think and respond to God any way I think appropriate. I know he is a big God." Such a reaction in essence is saying: "This is my world and my world has certain requirements by which it will run, and I am the one to set them. My world does not include this pain." Again the issue is one of control and resources.

Another mindset, the anesthetic principle, pictures the Bible and its answers as an anesthetic. Some people use biblical truth to numb the reality of the situation, protecting them from hurts. In this way, they don't have to deal with the reality of the situation. For example, consider this person's response to an incapacitating injury to a spouse: "Thank God for this tragedy because now I have more opportunity to serve my spouse." Or consider this mother's response to the sudden death of her child: "Praise God for taking my child. He wanted my baby to be with Him." On the surface, these responses sound good. But these persons often live out of a sense of duty, performing what he thinks is expected of them as believers. He thereby puts on hold, indefinitely or even permanently, the hard work of using the significant loss to grow and change. Or lastly, consider the patient with chronic pain: "God, me, and my faith have gotten me through it. If it weren't for Him and my faith, I wouldn't be here." He comforts himself that God will make it "all better." "Better" is defined as pain relief. More will be said about this under the theme of growing and changing in chapters 8 through 10.

But biblical truth is different. It was never designed to help people to avoid problems. The Bible presents a proper view, evaluation, and response to the realities of life. Three factors must be considered in order to accomplish God's goal of good stewardship. These are: the person in his circumstances, the God of life and those circumstances, and the nature of one's relationship to God. In 1 Samuel 30:1 through 8, we read how David was confronted with significant hardships of life. Finding his family and people carried off by the enemy, he wept until there was no strength left in him. His response was no different from his men in that respect. However, they became angry and lashed out at David, blaming him for their circumstances. On the other hand, David strengthened himself in the Lord and set to work. Unlike the world (1 Thessalonians 4:13), David had hope. This hope prevented his grief from moving toward despair because it was based, not on circumstances, but on the God of circumstances.

Paul's response to "I don't like" situations was the same as David's; they both knew and applied God's truth. Consider 2 Corinthians 1:8 through 10. Paul did not want the readers to be ignorant or misinformed about "how life treats us" (v. 8). In verse 9, he revealed the reason he wanted to inform the readers. It was so they would not rely on themselves but on God. The essence of life is a lordship issue: Is Jesus my boss, as well as my Savior? Will I submit to Him? Will I desire to be like Him, thereby pleasing God for Who He is and for what He has done for me in Christ? Or should I get what I want by having God at my beck and call? Am I going to function as the boss? Paul works out this theology throughout the book of 2 Corinthians (cf. 2 Corinthians 4:8–12; 6:3–12; 11:23–28; 12:7–10).

Jesus approached "I don't like" situations of life (in Jesus' case all of life was an "I don't like" situation!) in the same way.[a] Consider 1 Peter 2:23. What

---

a   There are many situations in life that are "I don't like" situations. For instance, the death of your spouse because of breast cancer (wife) or prostate cancer (husband). This is pressure from the outside. The key is your response and what motivates that response. There was much unpleasantness in Jesus' life. There were many things Jesus did not like: the money changers in the temple, the Pharisees misleading the sheep, and Peter's rebuke of Him recorded in Matthew 16:22. His dislike was not motivated by what was happening to Him (the circumstances of life). Rather, His dislike was a holy dislike motivated by a desire to uphold His Father's Name and honor. So did Jesus have "I don't like" situations? Was the cross one of them? The Bible says "yes." It gives us a view into the mind of Christ (Matthew 26:36–46; Mark 14:32–42; Luke 22:40–46; John 12:23–27). Jesus' response must be seen in the context of the big picture: the circumstances of Jesus' life were ordained by God in order to save a people for Himself and glorify the

the holy, harmless, undefiled One knew about His God and Father made the difference. Jesus actively, willfully, and cognitively called to mind those truths and therefore entrusted Himself into His Father's hands. The act of depositing or entrusting Himself to the Father resulted in returning good for evil by the cross (Romans 12:17–21).

Jesus deferred to His Father's will. He considered the "I don't like" situation as a blessing. Upon the cross, Jesus continued to return good for evil by ministering to unlovable people in an unlovely situation. Count the ways: He prayed for His executioners;[a] He evangelized the thief (Luke 23:39); He comforted His mother and John (John 19:25–27); and He remained on the cross accepting the full wrath of God in order to Honor the Father and the Triune God's eternal plan of redemption and to accomplish (John 6:37-43) and secure salvation for His people.

People think they do not deserve to be treated as God treated Jesus (Isaiah 53:4–6). Many people who have pain believe they deserve to be treated better than Jesus: "It was okay for Jesus to have His bodily problems, but not for me to have mine." In essence, some believe God should treat them better than He treated Jesus!

The anesthetic principle can also manifest itself when one is suffering. When it does, the sufferer takes center stage. Job did not think his suffering put him in a privileged position; even Paul wanted his suffering to end (2 Corinthians 12:7–10). In fact, Jesus considered asking the Father to remove the cup of the cross because of its heavy burden (John 12:23–27). Yet, some in the church exalt suffering and the "pain sufferer." Suffering is always the result of sin (Romans 5:12-14; 2 Corinthians 4;16-18). It may

---

Triune God. We know Jesus did not sin. John 4:34, using Jesus' own words, tells that He came to live among us: to do His Father's will. This He did because He was motivated to bring salvation to pass using the cross as His vehicle to do so.

a   Luke 23:34: this was not a prayer of blanket forgiveness, but a prayer in conformity to Mark 11:25. The Father answered that prayer with a "yes" at Pentecost.

be related to the person's individual and personal sin. However, it may be the result of being sinned against or simply part of God's sovereign plan. It is always a consequence of Adam's sin, God's judgment, and every person's except Christ, relationship to Adam (Romans 5:12-21).

Suffering, in and of itself, is neutral and colorless. It never brings about good. Rather, the response of the person in the midst of the suffering is what determines its value. Suffering exposes the heart of the matter – what happens in the inner man (James 4:1). One's inner allegiance is defined by what he really wants, desires, and seeks after. Fruit of this allegiance is expressed in his thinking and actions.

Consider the cross. Many people were crucified in Jesus' day. The cross was an instrument of death used by Rome as a deterrent. The person was humiliated to utmost degree and used to prevent any subordination against Rome. Jesus on the cross, not the cross alone, turns a person's understanding of pain and suffering upside down. How so? The curse of sin demanded a just, righteous God to act in a just manner. The guilt and condemnation for which Jesus suffered was the only fair outcome due to Adam's sin based on God's holiness, righteousness, and justice.

There are degrees of suffering, but in the end, no one can outrun the decaying of the outer man (2 Corinthians 4:16–18). Jesus, on the cross, dignified suffering. Although the purpose of the cross was redemption, "The cross dignified suffering by giving it meaning and demonstrated that it can have far-reaching effects for good."[71] Christ's death on the cross was the ultimate act of pleasing God rather than self. In His humiliation, and only in it as the Messiah, Jesus gave meaning to pain and suffering. He did not glorify it. Pain and suffering is due to sin, rebellion against and dissatisfaction with God. He did make it useful and even profitable as did his death on the cross. Because of the cross and a resurrected and ascended Savior, no believer should face trouble as an unbeliever does. It is sad when an unbeliever does take up the challenge of a failing body than the believer.

There is another side to this anesthetic principle approach to hard times. There is the belief that focuses on the "creative energy of God:" "The whole universe is full of it but only the amount of it that flows through our own beings will work for us." "We have tried often to make this creative power flow through us, saying 'Oh, God, please do this or that!'" "We doubt the willingness or ability of God to actually produce within our lives and bodies the results that we desire. We do not doubt our own ability to come into His presence and fill ourselves with Him, but His willingness to come into us and fill us with Himself."[72]

The author just quoted likens God to "the force" in the phrase "the force be with you." This phrase is taken from Stars Wars which is nothing more than New Age thinking and mysticism and "old age" mind over matter. God (or "the force") is spoken of as some impersonal, unseen agent. He is considered nothing more than cosmic energy that is willing or unwilling to enter a person and bring about healing. The author would have us believe that our job is to try and harness this energy by thinking of it as available to work through us. If this view of God is correct, then consider Job. In chapters 38 through 41 of that book, what is Job's response to God? Job's silence is deafening. Is Job's response in keeping with the previously quoted author's view of God? Certainly not! When Job finally does speak, it is in keeping with God as Creator (powerful, yet personal) and Job as a creature. Job humbled himself and then repented before God (Job 40:3–5, 42:1–6).

Read Genesis 1:1, 2; John 1:1–3; Colossians 1:15–18; or Hebrews 1:1–3 and 11:3. After reading those passages, ask yourself: How is it possible to make creative energy do something, much less harness and control it? Based on that author's view of God, it is easy to encourage people to use Him to bring about healing and change in conditions they do not like. God is likened to a "genie in the bottle." The bottle owner is greater than God. This view teaches that God does not say "no" to prayer. It teaches that God says "yes" only upon request, provided the person thinks about God and His willingness correctly. The bottom line is that the person controls God.

Finally, there is an approach to any "I don't like" situation, including pain and suffering to trouble and bodily problems that is fashioned after Kubler-Ross' so-called five stages of grief and acceptance.[73] She and others apparently think in terms of process, a change that occurs gradually. I hear patients speaking of "accepting," "coping," "facing it," and "coming to grips with what I have."

When I ask what all that means, patients say things such as: "A person needs time to process the new reality of pain." "It is hard to have a good outlook at first." "It may be helpful to allow for a time of grieving." "Accepting" seems to be living with the condition or disease and going on with life in spite of the disease or condition. One person commented that life was hard to face. When asked why, he reported: "Because dreams are shattered, hopes lost, and expectations are not met."

This "grief-work" mindset considers that one approach fits all: that everyone, when faced with an "I don't like" situation, will respond in a like manner. Further underlying this mindset is the belief that the person is not able to function when in an "I don't like" situation. His thinking will be impaired.

How did Jesus or any one of the heroes of faith mentioned in Hebrews 11 function? How did David respond when he and his men were faced with huge losses (1 Samuel 30:7), how did Job respond to the messengers' report and his wife's counsel (cf. Job 1:13–22; 2:10)? When a person is faced with trouble and one believes that an "acceptance" period is needed, biblical truth will not be considered as a worthy gift. If it is presented it will considered as a challenge not as a blessing.

Rather the person is left to his own resources. On this basis of this belief that there must be an "acceptance" period and during it, one is better off not being challenged by truth. Acceptance is usually defined as "getting used" to the "I don't like" situation, "learning to live with it," "coping," or simply "adjusting." This approach has no biblical basis.

Feelings, driven by unsatisfied and unfulfilled desires are often called "a sense of loss." These become authoritative driving forces. Futilely and seemingly forever, the person puts his energy into accepting his position. One person told me, "I am not Jesus or Paul." That patient considered himself relieved of any personal responsibility to develop Christlikeness. Life was a struggle and full of misery.

A corollary type of thinking includes the desire to have someone understand. Patients tell me: "I want you to know how badly I hurt." When asked why, often times they are not sure. Somehow they think that if "I (the physician) know," then something can be done to help them find pain relief. Perhaps the person is seeking assurance that things will be okay. Two co-authors write that when faced with adversity, "Our heartfelt plea is for assurance – fatherly assurance that there is an order to reality that transcends our problems, that somehow everything will turn out okay."[74]

There is a real and potential problem here. It centers on how one defines okay and by what means assurance is going to come. Okay must be defined according to biblical truth (see Genesis 50:19–21; Romans 8:28–39; and 2 Corinthians 5:9, 14–15). During hard times, it is easy to redefine okay to mean something other than what those passages teach It is easy to live the lie that things are out of control, have no good purpose, and that God has made a mistake.

When questioned further, patients often explain that their desire is to be understood and to have assurance from others. People can become objects and be used for one's own benefit. The seeker takes center stage and those around him are relegated to a servant's role.

Let me offer three other thoughts before we close this chapter. I have encountered patients who are waiting for and on God to use the pain for His glory. Such a person considers himself an innocent bystander. He is passive rather than actively, willfully, and cognitively using the situation as God's tool to grow and change (2 Corinthians 10:3-5). Consequently, he functions as a "couch potato" (see chapter 3). Another approach is the hope of being zapped whereby, without much (or any) effort on his part (except prayer), he will be instantly healed or removed from the "I don't like" situation.

Some think that only someone who has had a similar experience is able to minister to the person in need. What should be the response when someone says, "You haven't experienced what I have"? Behind that statement is the assumption that experience is superior to God's revealed truth. Or said another way: "What God has said is functionally inferior to my experience."

The truth is that believers do have One Who understands and knows (Hebrews 4:15; Isaiah 53:3). This One is the incarnate Christ, the Giver of all comfort. Who is interceding for the believer now (Romans 8:34; Hebrews 7:25). The Comforter is the same no matter what the situation or problem may be. Regardless of the problem, the comfort is the same because it is from God. He has so ordered things for believers that they may be able to comfort others in the same way He comforted His people (2 Corinthians 1:3–4). It is the Comforter and His comfort that are the key. In fact, the believer has two Comforters – Christ and the Holy Spirit (John 14:16-17, 26) Therefore the believer has all he needs to grow in Christlikeness no matter the situation or experience.

Questions that face every person are: What are your professed truths? and What truths do you live by? Put another way: Are your truths professed and confessed but functionally inoperative when faced with "I don't like" situations? With those questions before us and including the questions at the end of chapter 1, we are now ready to look at what God has to say in His Word regarding the subject of pain and bodily problems.

CHAPTER EIGHT

THE BIBLE: THE SOURCE OF GOD'S SUPERIOR ANSWER TO THE PROBLEM OF PAIN

UP TO THIS POINT, WE have reviewed what medicine, psychology, and the contemporary wisdom of society professes and uses. We have seen that there is an inordinate emphasis on pain relief. This thinking has no reference to good stewardship of the body (discussed in chapter 3). It leaves the person vulnerable to a constant pursuit of relief. A spirituality, not defined or described by the Bible, is included as an acceptable tool to achieve relief.

Further, with an emphasis on pain relief, a person's thinking will be colored by a self focus: "my resources to control my pain," "what others and situations and circumstances do that make my pain worse." The end result will be futile, even counterproductive. There is a price to be paid for this pursuit: bondage.

As I care for a patient, I attempt to discover what spiritual interests he has in solving problems. I want to know what his relationship to Christ is. If a patient is a believer, the next issue to discern is the impact of his relationship with Christ. If he is an unbeliever, I know he has no interest in solving problems God's way. Knowing where the patient is spiritually enables me to know where I must go and how to get there.

Sometimes patients, both believers and unbelievers, have no interest in bringing God's truth to bear on their problem of pain. I still care for them medically and minister to them. But I find that as I challenge a patient's thinking and wanting, changes may occur in how he "feels," including pain. Often, he reports less pain. In God's providence, the groundwork, then, has been prepared for me, to help move the patient toward a spiritual interest in solving problems using biblical truth.

What any person needs is something that gives reliable direction, guidance, and counsel. Why is counsel important? First, we were created to receive direction and counsel. We are counsel receivers just as Adam was before the fall. That being the case, the focus is on the source of the counsel. Is it from within (your own understanding, feelings and or experience and your interpretation of it) or from without (a source other than yourself)?

Most, if not all people, seek what they think is best. Most people who accept the wisdom of the culture usually define what is best for them as what makes them feel better, happy, and satisfied. Most patients who complain of pain usually define feeling better as pain relief. However, the evidence is clear that dissatisfaction, futility, and bondage characterize the life of the person who focuses on pain relief.

So, what is your source of wise counsel? If you owned a machine, where would you go to find out how it should work? If that machine didn't work properly, where would you go to find out how to repair it? In both cases, you should get out the owner's manual. Why? Because you know that the manual was written by the one who manufactured that equipment. The manufacturer has answers that you need. He is the one who knows.

So, where is the owner's manual for the problems of pain and bodies that don't work as you would like? You must go to the Creator and the Controller of His world. This is true for all areas of life. Not only did He create, He has provided an owner's manual, called the Bible. In it is God's superior answer to pain relief. Therefore, in regard to pain relief and all of life, you must seek wisdom from Scripture (Proverbs 2:1–8) and then apply it daily.

This chapter will look at a person's relationship to God (is he a believer or not?) and then his relationship to the Bible. A right relationship to God means the capacity for a right relationship to His Word. I see patients daily and I am struck by the fact that they (especially believers) demonstrate a lack of spiritual interest and understanding as it relates to their situations. As I have written, every person is a theologian. The issue is what kind is he.

Sometimes, patients never find God's superior answer. They may be unbelievers. Often, a believer responds as if he were unfamiliar with the Bible. When a patient pursues pain relief as his major goal in life, the curse of sin affects not only his body but his whole person, thinking and desires in the inner man and outer man. He has tried to match his thinking and wanting with God's yet he is dissatisfied and discontent. He is saying, in effect, he knows better than God. He is competing with God and God doesn't bless His competition (Isaiah 42:8; 48:11).

I shall attempt to convince you that the Bible has answers that are far superior to any wisdom of the age. As we study together, you will discover that God's superior answer brings Him glory and is best for you.

However, there is an initial problem. The answers in the Bible (God's owner's manual) are not for everyone. Why is that? Because not everyone is equipped to hear, accept, understand, and act on those answers.

They are unable to do so because not everyone has the proper receiving set to tune in to God's answers.

Any person can read the words in the Bible. These words are not similarly significant to all. In fact, many reject them (Romans 1:18-23) since they do not have the capacity to know, understand, and think spiritually (Matthew 11:25-27; Luke 10:20-22; 1 Corinthians 2:6-14). Their thoughts and ways are not God's (Isaiah 55:7-10). Why?

The problem is sin (Isaiah 59:1-2): not just one's own sin but his sin in Adam. The Bible clearly teaches that everyone born of a woman (except Christ) is reckoned to have sinned in Adam[a] and is therefore guilty before God (Romans 3:9-19, 23; 5:12-21). In Adam, he is condemned and liable for God's punishment. If nothing changes, misery in this life and in the next is the only outcome. This representative principle, by which Adam represented all men, is similar to the system in the United States whereby an elected official represents his constituents.

A person is not only guilty (liable for punishment) and condemned, but he is also corrupt. This means because he is a sinner, he sins. By nature, orientation, and instinct, he is a self-pleasing, anti-God rebel.

Sadly, most people deny these facts. He is on one side of the fence where only the answers of contemporary wisdom are available to him. These answers compound the misery of life. Yet, God in His mercy and

---

a   Adam, and therefore man, was created after God's own image, upright, in knowledge, holiness, and righteousness (Genesis 1:26-27; Ecclesiastes 7:29; Ephesians 4:24; Colossians 3:10). We and the rest of mankind are joined to Adam, representatively, so that what Adam was and did is counted to us. That is, as Adam was in the garden, so we were in the garden. What Adam did, we did. When Adam sinned, he lost his original righteousness, was guilty and under condemnation, and there was a corruption of his whole nature. Since we are in Adam, this loss of original righteousness, guilt, condemnation, and corruption are counted to us and all mankind. Therefore, being in Adam means that we are sinners (guilty and condemned, having a corrupt and polluted nature) and therefore we sin (because of our corrupt, polluted nature). This in no way relieves any person of responsibility for his sin. We cannot blame Adam, the devil, or God Himself (James 1:13-15).

grace offers His answers. These answers are announced by the Word:
the living Word, Jesus Christ (John 14:6), and the written word, the
Bible (John 17:17). Jesus alone is the gate that leads to the other side of
the fence (John 10:1–10).

There is no other way (Acts 4:12). Those on one side are without
God's answers, in bondage, and given over to the futility of human
wisdom and desires (Ephesians 4:17–19). The other side of the fence is
the place where God's answers to all problems in this life may be found.
These answers include how to evaluate and respond to God and His
providence. A proper vertical reference and orientation leads to proper
thinking about God, the person's condition, and the proper response..

God always has you and me right where He wants us. He is a Sovereign God. Assume with me that human answers have lost their appeal.
The futility of seeking to be free of pain or relatively pain-free has become burdensome. You, or some other person you know, have grown
weary and tired of the struggle. So what now? More of the same? No.
You, or he, may well be ready for God's counsel and guidance.

How does one move to the side of the fence where he can find and
apply the answers of the Bible? Only in one way: through a living,
intimate, personal relationship with Jesus Christ. This relationship
ushers in trusting in, depending upon, and applying biblical truth
as a new creature in Christ indwelt by the Holy Spirit. The relationship is established by the Holy Spirit and is called regeneration or
rebirth. Better it is a supernatural birth from heaven (John 3:3-8). It
means salvation. It means that an invader God[a] has chosen in His

---

a   The term *invade* can mean entering and even intruding in unwanted and even
unwelcomed places for the purpose of doing harm and plundering. The term, *invader
God*, pictures the first aspect of the meaning. Certainly, the unbeliever opposes and
resists God. Romans 5:6–10 and 8:5–8 describe man's condition of hostility, rebellion,
and resistance to God. Yet, God chooses to enter into a relationship with such a person,
not for the purpose of doing evil but for the purpose of doing good.

mercy and compassion to do radical heart surgery to those whom He causes to believe.

The result of that "surgery" is a supernatural transformation that only God can bring about (John 3:3-8; Ezekiel 36:26). This transformation is the new birth which results in a new creation (2 Corinthians 5:17). This new life is implanted into previous enemies, rebels, and strangers who lived on the side of the fence (Ephesians 2:1-6) Then and only then is the person able to listen to the gospel call and turn to God and away from his previous manner of thinking and behavior, thereby becoming part of a new kingdom (Colossians 1:13).

So what is this relationship and how does it come about? Relationships occur between persons. The Bible clearly teaches that God is a Person, a thinking, moral Being, and that man is made in His image. From the beginning, man was made to be in relationship to Him. This relationship and communion depended on Adam's righteous life before God. He was on probation and could forfeit that relationship and communion, and exchange it for another: a relationship with the world, self, and Satan.[a] When Adam sinned, sin entered the world and separated people from God. They are guilty, condemned, and are unable not to sin.

Yet, this is God's world, and He is not Someone you can take or leave at a whim. No, He is the Creator of the universe, the Author and Giver of life itself. Being out of relationship to God means to be in relationship to self as a pleaser of self, to the ideas and values of the world as a system of thought and behavior opposed to God, and to Satan.

---

a   The word *probation* indicates the testing or trial of a person. The test or trial may be brought about because the person has something counted against him but is not yet imprisoned. This was not the case with Adam. Adam had perfect righteousness and was given the command not to eat of the fruit to prove the genuineness of this righteousness.

In contrast, being in relationship to God means being complete in Christ. This completeness has to do with how God reckons or accounts your life. God did this in eternity past (Ephesians 1:4–6, 11; Revelation 3:5; 13:8; 17:8). The result of this reckoning is that each one of His people is counted perfect and complete in His Son. There is still the matter of the daily living out of that perfection; believers are counted perfect in Christ even though their practice doesn't agree with God's reckoning. At times, the believer functions as an unbeliever does.

What does it mean then to be "a new creation" in Christ (2 Corinthians 5:17)? It means several things. Creation implies that because something supernatural was done, there was a supernatural result. That is exactly what rebirth is all about. Rebirth, birth from above,or regeneration means that a person's state or condition has been changed, radically, from the inside out so that a new way of thinking, wanting, and acting results.

Previously, that person, as an unbeliever, had a wrong standing before God. He had been judged condemned and guilty before God. Now his record is seen before God as spotless (Isaiah 1:18). God is a bookkeeper, par excellence, and He has made a radical change on His ledger sheet. He has taken that person's unrighteousness and placed it on the ledger of the only perfect person, Jesus Christ. He took Christ's righteousness and right standing before Himself, Christ's very Father, and placed that on the person's ledger sheet. Now when God in His justice looks at the person's ledger and judges according to what that person has and has not done, He sees only a right standing for that person because of the double transfer He brought about. In God's amazing justice and love, the One who justifies is the One who saves (Romans 3:21–26)! All of this comes about because the believer is "in

Christ"; he has been brought into communion with God. God is no longer his enemy.

But that is not all! Not only does the believer obtain a new state (new birth) and a right standing (new record), but also a change in status. This status change means that the saved person has been transferred into God's family (adoption). He has been adopted (Romans 8:14–23; 9:4; Galatians 4:5; Ephesians 1:5) with all the rights and privileges that come with it. He has a source of reliable, authoritative, and kind counsel and guidance.

Based on the Bible's teaching and counsel and has the believer moves darkness to light, he realizes that the goal is not to get relief. It is to have victory in the midst of trouble. That is one of the lessons of the cross. The believer is already counted a victor because he is in Christ, the Victor (Romans 9:35-39). The believer is called to close the gap between what he is in Christ by God's reckoning and what he is in practice. The misery of this world becomes his workshop and even his tool (Philippians 2:12–13; 2 Peter 1:10).

What does all the above mean for one's pain and bodily problems? We will discuss this at length in chapter 13 as we apply the principles we are learning. Suffice it to say here, a right relationship with God through Jesus Christ is the cornerstone to being a victor in the midst of painful times. Being a victor in tough times means thinking and responding as Christ did. It means developing Christlikeness as a privilege and blessing not simply out of duty (1 John 3:1-3).

Once rebirth has occurred, a person is indwelt by the Holy Spirit (Romans 5:5) Who gives to the believer a new capacity to desire the things of God, to understand His word, and to act accordingly. The person's relationship with Christ and the indwelling Holy Spirit as

Christ's guarantee and surety (Ephesians 1:13–14, 3:16-21) makes all the difference in the world. How?

The person now has the right receiving set, he is on the right side of the fence. He desires to understand the owner's manual and apply it to the problems of pain.

The believer is counted perfect in his state by regeneration, in his standing by justification through faith, and in his family status by adoption and through the indwelling of the Holy Spirit (John 14:16–17, 26; 15:26). Believers still sin; they are perfect in Christ in principle but not yet in practice. Their thinking and ways in daily life are not consistently God's thoughts and ways. They do not act as perfected creatures. Sinful patterns remain. This includes the lack of application of biblical principles in responding to pain and bodily problems God's way. Yet, this need not be. There is hope. The Bible provides what the believer needs for his life after salvation (2 Peter 1:3–4; 2 Timothy 3:15–17). God's Word simplifies life by giving clear, consistent, and refreshing direction from the outside. Living life God's way takes the person off the merry-go-round of feeding wants, hopes, expectations, desires, and goals.

What in the Bible is better and superior to pain relief? Simply put, it is being satisfied and content with God and your salvation even when pain relief is not possible or does not come. It is satisfaction and contentment (even joy) that comes from pleasing God with a body that does not always work , or function as one desires even demands. It is using unpleasantness and daily discomfort to become more like Christ. It is understanding and accepting God's goodness in the situation and responding in a God-honoring way by growing and changing so as to become more like Christ.

You may be wondering: If that is all there is to it, how is this better than pain relief? Fair enough. The answer to your question is found in the Bible. We must go back to the beginning. But what beginning? Paul begins before creation in eternity past, before the foundation of the world (John 6:37-43; Ephesians 1:3–14; also see Revelation 3:5; 13:8; 17:8).

These verses are the Holy Spirit's commentary on God's original design. Paul, in Ephesians, likely his circular letter to the churches in Asia Minor, takes the saints to heavenly places (Ephesians 1:3). Only the triune God was there. Paul praises God the Father for being the God and the Father of Jesus Christ. He then begins to record and catalogue a series of divine gifts, the first being God's blessing of all the saints with every spiritual blessing in the heavenly realm (Ephesians 1:3).

The ultimate blessing any believer can receive is Jesus Christ Himself and the indwelling of the Holy Spirit. Since the triune God was the only one present in eternity past (before the foundation of the world), it is obvious that salvation is of the Lord. It is 100% His work.

In Ephesians 1:4, Paul speaks of the saints being chosen (or called out) from among the nations. How are the saints chosen? They are chosen in Christ – that is the thrust of Paul's list of spiritual blessings. He does His choosing by establishing a relationship between Himself and believers. He does this by placing the believer in Christ.

What were the saints chosen for? Paul describes life after salvation this way: to be holy and blameless (Ephesians 1:4). Now, what do these terms mean? Holy means set apart from something to something, and blameless means without internal defect, blemish, or spot. Simply put, all believers are to be like Jesus Christ, the only Person Who always pleased God (Matthew 3:17; 17:5). God the Father thought so well of His

Son that He intended every believer to be like Him. This was God's design before salvation and it is His design after salvation.

Are you beginning to see the connection? To be "in Christ" makes all the difference: What is Christ's is yours. His victory is your victory. His preeminent position, at the right hand of the Father, is your position as well (Colossians 3:1-3). You no longer know God only as Judge, but also as Father. You have a place of refuge, security, and shelter. These truths are to be hidden in your heart (Psalm 119:9-11) in order to be brought to mind and recalled when days get long and pain seems endless. They are the stepping stones for gaining victory in the midst of hard times.

God's purpose in making mankind and in recreating fallen man as believers was to make them like Christ. Only then would they be able to enter into and to enjoy the presence of God. Only then would God's eternal purpose be fulfilled – a people for Himself in worship and fellowship.Man's chief end is to know God and enjoy Him forever. He was made by Him and for Him (Romans 11:33–36; Colossians 1:15–18; Revelation 4:11). Thus, man can glorify God only when he is in Christ and becoming more like Christ.

For any person to fulfill his chief end in life, he must do what he has been designed by God to do: to live like Christ. Being like Christ is a matter of pleasing God. That is what Jesus did and that is what each of God's saints has been designed to do (Ephesians 1:3–4). When a person's goal is to become like Christ and please God, he can be compared to a train on the track rather than in the water trying to be a boat or the airplane in the sky rather than on the road trying to drive like a car. Both train and airplane will be destroyed if used improperly. However, both operate smoothly when in their proper spheres. The same is true of people. Not only is it delightful and satisfying for a person to live the way God designed him; but it is also the only way for him (or anyone) to live a satisfying, delightful life.

You still may be wondering: How is Christlike living better than pain relief – especially when it hurts so much? This is a good question. We have learned that pain relief is not guaranteed in this life. We know that God has not chosen to reverse the curse of sin on the body (2 Corinthians 4:16–18). We also have seen that while it is not necessarily wrong to pray for pain relief, God may say "no," "wait a while," or "I have something better."

However, since the believer is in Christ, becoming more like Christ in this life is a reality, not yet fully realized. It is always possible to grow so as to please God. When a person is living to please God, he is becoming more like Christ.

What are the results? God is delighted and the person is delighted (he should be!). Consider that in light of a day in my office. Day after day, I meet patients who are "unhappy campers." They are discouraged and upset and anything but delighted (and delightful). Their goal is pain relief which has been elusive. When pain relief is the person's goal pleasing the Father can't be. Pleasing the Father is much the same as pleasing your earthly parent. There is a certain satisfaction and contentment that results. That is part of the fresh breeze I mentioned at the end of chapter 5. Satisfaction in this life can come despite any situation or person. Satisfaction (even contentment) comes despite the pain!

Life is simplified, goals and direction are clear, and one's hope is not some "hope so" hope because it is solidly rooted in his relationship with Christ. This means that living out that relationship is far more important than getting something from God. In this life no one can outrun the curse of sin including pain and bodily problems.

A Christian's God-given joy, which is Jesus Himself, cannot be taken away by the circumstances including hard times no matter what they may be (John 16:20–22). Consequently, the believer will use what seems to be very bad for God's purpose of perfecting and maturing his relationship with Christ.

This scenario contrasts with a "hope so" approach to life which leaves patients at the mercy of their situation, hoping against hope that pain will leave for an extended period of time, and that the body will be restored.

Consider Psalm 37:23–24:

> *If the Lord delights in a man's way, he makes his steps firm;*
> *though he stumble, he will not fall, for the Lord upholds him*
> *with His right hand.*

Living in a body that doesn't work as well as one would like is taxing. A painful body is generally one that is inefficient. More energy is required to perform tasks. Bones and joints don't move by themselves. Bodily movement is the role of the soft tissue of the body, in particular, muscles and tendons. When joints are abnormal, the back is out of proper alignment, and or muscles are deconditioned (which occurs in any number of disorders), then muscles are called to function in ways for which they were not designed.

I explain this to patients this way: "Your body is functioning as a pulley in need of grease. It will get the job done but it takes more energy to do so." Or I may say: "Your body is like a 1960 Ford and will probably never be the newest model Ford. Yet, if you drive carefully and maintain it, it will serve you." These patients have found out that there are daily ups and downs in regard to the functioning of their bodies and how they feel.

So what sustains them? Sometimes, nothing. Sometimes, it is only the hope of a little relief. Either way the downward spirit of pain and more pain continues. In contrast, the passages before us clearly point out that though there are daily ups and downs, God's hand is steady. Circumstances may change, but God does not. He is the God of circumstances. Since God does not change, then your joy and delight need not. God is steady and what He provides is more than sufficient for you to honor Him. God will sustain! Therefore, the believer is to be a Galatians 2:20 person. Paul said that it is not the old person who lives but Christ Who lives in him (the new I) and helps him live a new life of faith. The new I lives the new life of saving faith. Paul makes this point in 2 Corinthians 4:16–18. The curse of sin has resulted in a decaying body, but for the believer, the inner man is being renewed. Renewal of the inner man means maturing in faith and growing and changing as one develops more of the character of Christ.

This takes us back to where we began: to God's original design before the foundation of the world. The believer's changed thinking, wanting, and behavior result from the fulfillment of God's original design to make man like Christ by placing him in Christ by the Holy Spirit. This God-established and Holy Spirit-sustained relationship leads to growth Christlikeness, a desire to please God, and actually pleasing God in all situations.

Do you see how a changed relationship between you and God gives a whole new perspective on the fact of pain? If not, I suggest you study again what it means to be "in Christ" and how that relationship changes the way one thinks about life including pain. Consider Psalm 1:1–3:

> Happy is the man who does not walk in the counsel of the
> wicked or stand in the way of sinners or sit in the seat of

mockers. But his delight is in the law of the Lord, and on his law he meditates day and night, he is like a tree planted by streams of living water, which yields its fruit in season and whose leaf does not wither. Whatever he does prospers.

There you have it: God clearly points out that a worthwhile life comes about when one is living and as Jesus modeled during His time as the Messiah. This is what all believers have been re-created to do. Pleasing God was Jesus' satisfaction and it is to be the believers' who are in Christ.

A New Testament commentary on these passages is given in 2 Corinthians 5:9: "So we make it our goal to please Him, whether we are at home in the body or away from it." This verse should never be separated from verse 15 in which Paul tells his readers "that those who live should no longer live for themselves but for Him who died for them and was raised again." Again, Paul describes the results of God's radical heart surgery: believers are changed into people who no longer live to get what they want, but to please God.

How is it possible to be what a person was designed to be and become like Christ? How is it possible to please God when my body hurts? How is this satisfying and even delightful? The answer is in terms of relationships. It is possible one way only – through a personal, close, intimate relationship with Jesus Christ as Lord and Savior. Moreover, as a child of God, the believer is indwelt with the Holy Spirit and he is surrounded by fellow believers who are in Christ and indwelt by the Holy Spirit (Ephesians 4:11- 14) Being "in Christ" is salvation which opens the way to live as one saved!. The believer is then on the right side of the fence and in a position to find and appropriate God's help. Being in Christ is essential for thinking, desiring, and acting as a God-pleaser.[a]

A believer has spiritual life after salvation. Look at what the believer has been saved from: the wrath of God, the sting of death, the condemnation and guilt of sin, the power of sin, the curse of perfect, personal lawkeeping as the means of salvation, himself, and bondage to Satan. Moreover, the believer also has been saved to something. He is saved to a life of becoming more like Christ. This means daily dying to self, which is done by growing and changing and developing the character of Christ in thoughts, desires, and actions (Matthew 10:32–39; 16:24–25; Mark 8:31–37; Luke 9:23–26; 14:26–28; John 12:25). Life with all its ups and downs is the stage on which the believer develops a growing and maturing relationship with Jesus Christ. Being "in Christ" means each believer is given resources to grow and change. Living out that relationship is of such importance that God has made equipping saints a major function of the church (Ephesians 4:11–16). It was a major purpose of Paul's ministry (Colossians 1:28).

---

a   Believers are both saved and are being saved. Both facts result from being "in Christ." The believer is saved "in Christ" as his state, record, status, and capacity are perfect because he is in Christ. God cannot, nor can Jesus Himself, bring a charge against God's elect because they are perfect in Christ (Romans 8:32–34; Hebrews 7:25). Paul expresses the fact of salvation in terms of being dead to sin as Jesus died to sin once for all (Romans 6:10–11). He exhorts his readers to remember this fact. Paul, writing under the inspiration of the Holy Spirit, thinks it is important for the saints to know the fact of being "in Christ." This knowledge is to motivate a believer to live out his salvation (life after salvation) becoming more and more like Christ. Paul discusses this in Romans 6–8.

CHAPTER NINE

MORE OF THE
BIBLE'S SUPERIOR ANSWER
FOR PAIN

THE BIBLE VIEWS PAIN AS a given. Given, universal, and inescapable. It is part of life in a fallen world (Genesis 3:16–19; Romans 5:12–24; 2 Corinthians 4:16–18). Contrary to what one patient told me, this truth does not mean it is acceptable to respond to bodily problems sinfully. Frustration, worry, anger, and fear are common expressions. The signal the core issues of control and resources. They are based on a person's thinking about the self. Pain is the result of God's curse on sin. The fact that individuals experience pain does not necessarily mean that the individual is a greater sinner than others or that he is receiving his "just due."

In truth, every person deserves the worst kind of pain. Most people don't believe that fact or only give lip service to it. Why does every person deserve pain? Proper theology is needed to answer this question. Now you know why it was important to discuss our union with Adam at length in chapter 8. What is the worst kind of pain? It is hell and eternal separation from God. The unbeliever has a taste of hell on the earth. He is separated from God and the misery of this life apart from God is foretaste of hell. Luke 16:19-31 depicts this final separation as complete and irreversible. Revelation 20:10 gives a vivid description of this worst pain:

> *And the devil who deceived them was thrown into the lake*
> *of burning sulfur where the beast and the false prophet had*
> *been thrown. They will be tormented day and night for ever*
> *and ever.*

The picture here is of torment. The word carries the meaning "torture, afflict, vex, toss about, and harass." This condition can be compared to a movie without an intermission or end. The lake of fire burns but is never extinguished. One can almost smell the stench of burning sulfur. Yet the burning never ends. Not even death itself, by whatever means (including assisted suicide), can remove you from this forever and forever-ness. It is the worst kind of misery that anyone will ever experience.

In this life, pain comes from the reasons given in chapter 3. Physical illness and pain are not necessarily caused by a person's specific sin. If you have pain now or in the future, this truth may well apply to you. This is shown clearly in the life of Job and also in the man born blind in John 9.

The Bible is the authority when pain and responding to pain are the issues. And because bodily problems are part of this life, the issue is not between pain and no pain. Rather, the issue is how one will respond to the body he has whether there is pain or not. A response to God's providence is a response to God. Your response depends upon your theology. That means it is imperative to study the Bible to learn God's truth.

The Bible's superior answer to pain relief is quite simple but not simplistic (see chapter 8). It is being satisfied and contented even when pain relief and freedom from bodily problems don't come. There are no guarantees in this life in terms of pain relief. God's truth helps you to be motivated and even excited about being satisfied, regardless of pain relief. God's knowledge and ways take guessing out of tough times. It is the ultimate answer to any "why?" or "why me?" questions that you could ask. The result is a simplified life that is refreshing. You will be able to focus on pleasing God and not on pain relief.

God's answer is simple, not "simplistic" (which implies inadequacy because of a lack of complexity). Rather, Jesus Christ, the God-man, reveals the unfathomable and complex Being of the Triune God Who is God Himself (Colossians 1:15-18, John 1:18). Therefore, through Jesus, the believer is able to relate to the Creator God, the just God, and the Redeemer-Savior God in an intimate way. Jesus bids His people to come to Him and receive rest (Matthew 11:28–30). Jesus' call is not simply evangelistic. Personal lawkeeping highlighted the religion of Israel. As a result, the people were heavy burdened. They desired something from God and tried the keep laws, theirs in place of God's. Lovingly yet firmly Jesus wooed the people to come to Him, learn from Him and about Him and rely on His lawkeeping. Similarly seeking pain relief to get so often burdens the believer.

Jesus' invitation (it is actually a summons) addressed the principle of salvation by works. Jesus' answer turned people from the bondage of law-keeping as an end in itself to the source of genuine relief. He was the source of their rest. He had come to set His people free. This new principle applies not only to salvation but to life after salvation. The genuine relief that Jesus speaks about is summed up as growing and changing.

Paul writes (2 Corinthians 5:9, 14–15) that the love of God, in Christ, compels (or funnels) him along to one conclusion: he cannot live for himself and his own satisfaction. The love of God and his knowledge and love of it so motivated him to please God that he could not live for himself and his own satisfaction. Seeking to please God[a] is God's way of satisfaction and contentment for him and all believers. Any other way is bondage to sin, Satan, and self.

When you don't get what you want or think is best for you, or if you do, what is your source of satisfaction and contentment? It should be your relationship with Christ. Recognizing what you are in Christ is the way to use the pain to grow and change and to develop the willingness to be satisfied and contented.

Part of the lesson presented in the Old Testament relating to the Levitical system of clean and unclean was the constant choice placed before each Israelite. It was a " . . . means of alerting the Jew to the fact that all day long, every day, in whatever he does, he must consciously choose God's way."[b][75] So it is for every believer when daily faced with pain: to choose to use (or not use) what he does not like to grow and change in Christlikeness. Again this is one of the lessons of the cross (1 Corinthians 1:18-31).

---

a   In John 4:31–34, Jesus contrasted His source of satisfaction and contentment (pleasing His Father) to the source with which the disciples were more familiar: the pleasure of eating. They sensed delight and pleasure after eating. Jesus was satisfied and contented with pleasing God. His desire to do the will of His Father resulted from His relationship with Him. The results of Jesus pursuing any other way of satisfaction would be incredible, almost unbelievable. Jesus would not have accomplished His mission and He would have been a dissatisfied God-man. Heaven forbid!

b   Paul gloried and exulted about his weaknesses, especially his bodily problems. Why? His theology was correct. He knew that when he was devoid of his own wisdom and strength, God had him right where He wanted him. He was forced to be dependent on God and wise in God's eyes rather than in his own strength and wisdom (2 Corinthians 12:7–10).

Since this is God's world, all is His. He has entrusted everything to believers and expects a return. The issue is not stewardship or no stewardship, but what kind of steward you are: good or bad? The person who seeks only pain relief as a primary goal will not take care of other parts of his body. Consider the diabetic who will not follow his diet, the emphysema patient who refuses to stop smoking, or the patient with a rheumatic condition who chooses not to exercise. The desire for pain relief, when apart from good stewardship, neglects taking care of the entire body. This is an example of bad stewardship. Why?

Pain relief as a primary goal focuses on the inferior goal of what the person wants (pain relief). This takes attention away from what God is doing and desires the believer to think, desire, and do in the situation. What is God's intention and purpose in running His world His way? He brings various situations into the believer's life for any number of reasons. It is His superior goal for the believer to use this situation to become more like Christ. This principle applies in instances of both acute pain (example: headache) and chronic pain (examples: RA or fibromyalgia). If you simply want to relieve your headache, you will reach for pain medication without a thought of using this situation to become more like Christ. This may be failing to redeem the "time" (situation) for growing and changing (Ephesians 5:15–18). The "how to's" for redeeming the time are discussed in chapter 13.

On the other hand, to refrain from taking medication or even seeking a diagnosis, may also be bad stewardship. Patients tell me: "I don't want to take anything if I can help it." When asked why, they say: "I don't like taking medications. I don't want to get hooked on them." What is going on in their thinking? What is motivating them? This is not always easy for me to know. In seeking to know, sometimes I discover it is the cost of the medication. Sometimes, it is fear. Sometimes, the patient simply doesn't like or think he deserves what he has, and by not taking something is proof he isn't in the situation.

The reason is not as important as helping the patient see that taking or not taking medication is not the issue. Neither is it pain or no pain. The issue is growing and changing and using the situation for doing that.

Christlikeness, then, should be the goal of all believers. Christlikeness focuses on what God is doing and wanting to accomplish in and through the situation. What God is doing is also best for the individual believer. How so? Consider the ultimate human experience. What is it? It is seeing God face to face. That is what is promised to all believers (1 John 3:1–3). John placed this "seeing" in the context of family. John was amazed at the profound radical transfer from one family and kingdom to another (Colossians 1:13). John begins by reflecting on God's amazing love. Why this reflection? Believers were adopted, brought into, God's family. God, the Judge, declaring sinners not guilty nor condemned was a great thing. Yet, that's not all – that same Judge now takes the person home as His son. To John, that was truly amazing.

The picture in these verses reminds me of a family union. There is great anticipation for the coming get-together and the joy associated with the event itself. In fact, John tells us that the hope and anticipation of that great event are what motivates people to purify themselves in this life (v. 3). This is John's way of describing growing and changing.

Throughout the Old Testament, the thought of seeing God was frightening and even thought to bring death (Genesis 16:13; 32:30; Exodus

24:10–11; 33:20, 23; Judges 6:22; 13:22). Yet John, in the New Testament (1 John 3:1–3), writes that this is exactly what believers are promised. How does one reconcile these two thoughts?

In the Old Testament, God revealed Himself to individuals but never fully. In Exodus 33:18 and following, Moses asked God to show him His glory. In the previous verse, God had told Moses: "I am pleased with you and I know you by name." Moses had God's approval. In His approval, God basically said that I consider you in the same way as I consider my yet-to-come Son. We know this is the case because Jesus Christ was the only Person about Whom God thought well (Matthew 3:17; 17:5).

Moses was God's mediator between God and His people. Moses represented God's people to God and God to His people. In this way, Moses prefigured Christ, the greater Moses. Moses was to function in the same manner as Christ did but Moses never went to the cross. He did not bear the wrath of God. He did point to Jesus and highlighted the fact that God must be approached through someone God has chosen as His agent to bring his people to him. Jesus by focusing on pleasing the Father rather Himself was preparing to be the better and the mediator of a better covenant. Jesus stayed the course, again, not out of duty but because of His earnest desire to please the Father (Hebrews 2:10; 5:8; 3:1- 6; 8:1-13; 10:1-4, 19-25). So, too, Moses. He had to follow in Jesus' footsteps. Moses was to grow individually but also as God's mediator. Moses' growth pointed to God's glory. How else would it be possible for anyone to please God unless God established a relationship with him?

Yet God chose to hide Himself. Why? Because Moses could not stand in God's presence and live – nor can we unless one is in Christ. Ultimately that waits heaven. God put Moses in the cleft of the rock, nestled in its safety (Exodus 33:22). Where is the best place for that safety and security? The Bible pictures both God and Jesus as the Rock (Deuteronomy 32:4, 15, 18, 30–31; 1 Corinthians 10:4). Figuratively speaking, Moses was placed "in Christ." Moses was not there yet in terms of his Christlikeness. By placing him in the cleft of the rock, God was growing and maturing Moses through His relationship with Moses. As a result, Moses could look forward to the ultimate blessing that results from his relationship with God: seeing God face to face (1 John 3:1–3).

Believers will not see God face to face in this life; that awaits our entrance into heaven. Yet, just as Moses did, we have a piece of that experience right now. How so? The next best human experience to seeing God face to face in heaven is becoming more like Christ in this life. True freedom is for the believer to become what he was designed to be. As he grows and changes, the believer benefits because he avoids the way of the transgressor, the unfaithful one, fool (Proverbs 13:15b; 26:11). God's glory and the good of the individual believer are inextricably bound together. They are inseparable. That is great news for those in the trenches, daily facing pain.

In the case of pain, Christlikeness develops in at least three ways. First, as you use your body to please God even when it doesn't always work as you want, or feel as you want, this becomes a blessing to you (Philippians 4:13). I will develop this in chapter 13. People say "I can't" because it hurts. When I ask them if they are paralyzed, they most often answer "no." Some will say "I can't move," but in fact they refuse to move in order to avoid pain.

If the believer is correct in his assumption that his body won't allow him to function, then what is he saying? If God's design for him is to be like Christ, he is saying he can't fulfill God's design. Further, he is saying that God made a mistake by giving him a body that won't let him accomplish God's purposes for him on earth. Further still, he is saying that Paul and the Holy Spirit are wrong (see Romans 8:35–37 and 2 Corinthians 12:7–10).

Second, Christlikeness also develops as you respond to pain and the lack of pain relief by using the daily discomfort and unpleasantness of your life as God's agents of change (Philippians 1:12–18). Paul did not think it "bad" or "wrong" or a "bad deal" that he was in prison. Paul responded to his restrictions (Roman prison and his wrists chained to a guard) by looking down the chain at the other end and seeing a captive guard. Why? Paul's theology included using situations, especially hard times, to bring about Christlikeness in himself, in part, by ministering to others. How did he do this? He sought to learn what God was doing in the problem. He understood that the problem was bigger than himself, but not bigger than God. He desired to serve God by serving others. He therefore concluded that his "prison" was really a church, and the guard, a person to befriend and evangelize.

Third, Christlikeness also develops when you use the body God gave you for God's glory, no matter how damaged or disappointed in it you are (Genesis 45:5ff.; 50:19–21; Romans 8:28–29). For now, I am speaking of the motivation behind that "using."

The believer's theology is crucial: his understanding of Who God is and what He brings about. Correct theology means that the believer acknowledges God's intention and purpose for him to use unpleasantness to become more like Christ. He accepts that God is a good, wise God. He then applies this truth in his daily life. He realizes this is best for him and most glorifying to God.

Christlikeness is God's purpose for every believer. In one sense, Christlikeness has happened. The believer has a new identity (he is in Christ and Christ's perfection has been reckoned to him) and with that identity comes a radical change in his goal, his agenda to reach it, and his efforts to pursue it. In another sense, Christlikeness is still happening. How that happens will be the subject of the next chapter.

CHAPTER TEN

BECOMING MORE LIKE CHRIST: THE PURPOSE OF THE BELIEVER'S RELATIONSHIP WITH CHRIST

IN CHAPTERS 8 THROUGH 9, the truth was exposed that satisfaction and contentment in this life come from pleasing God. Contrary to the wisdom of the age, there is no other source. To find out why, let's review what we have learned. (1) Every believer is designed to be in Christ for the purpose of pleasing God; (2) Believers are able to please God because they are in relationship to Him in Christ; (3) Being able to be what one is designed to be is true freedom; (4) True freedom is a source of hope, endurance, and joy; (5) It is best for the believer to follow God's design for him; and (6) It is futile, even counterproductive, to live otherwise.

Being saved, a past event, also means doing daily what God has designed, a present event. Therefore, becoming more like Christ is the very essence of the Christian life.

However, not everyone has been taught this truth, nor do they necessarily understand it even if they have read it or heard it. Many believers think that life after salvation is focused on what the person has become in Christ rather than how to become more like Christ in his daily life. When the focus is on the past event of salvation, the past event of salvation, the Christian life is considered a "done deal," and the believer assumes a passive role in it. That is, he doesn't appreciate or acknowledge his responsibility in the growing process. There is little emphasis on encouraging active daily growing and changing using the problems of life as God's tools for developing Christlikeness. Rather, the Christian life is characterized by a "let go and let God" mentality. The cry is something like this: "I don't try to change myself. I rely on the Holy Spirit to do that." Or "I just preach the gospel to myself."

Thinking this way is the result of a failure to understand and act upon the Bible's teaching regarding biblical change. That teaching can be summarized by correctly answering the question: Who produces sanctification – the Holy Spirit or the believer? The answer is both. While regeneration is monenergistic - 100% the work of the holy Spirit and 0% of the person- progressive sanctification is 100% God and 100% the believer. The Holy Spirit works in and with the believer but never for or against the believer. Change (sanctification) occurs when the believer obeys the Bible through the power of the Holy Spirit. Progressive sanctification involves the whole in terms of changed thinking and desires which leads to God-pleasing actions. Emphasizing either the believer's responsibility or the Spirit's work to the exclusion of the other is wrong. Rather, there is a double contribution to the process of change. The believer (not the Spirit) obeys through the grace given to him by the Holy Spirit.[76]

If the believer fails to understand and act upon the Bible's teaching regarding biblical change, the problems of life, rather than God's solutions, take center stage. If such a believer, who is in Christ, hasn't been taught that the truth of God's Word applies to solving and overcoming the problems of life, then he is tempted to seek "something more" instead of "more of the something" that he is in Christ.

To be in Christ in principle is an instantaneous act done to the believer by God Himself. But life after salvation is a becoming more like Christ in practice. Progressive sanctification is a growing reality in the life of a believer who is now able to think God's thoughts, desire God's desires, and follow God's commands. In short, he trusts and obeys, applying biblical principles to the problems of life including pain and bodily problems.

In addition, some have difficulty accepting and acting on the fact that something so bad (or something that feels so bad) as pain, can be good or used for good. It is common, almost natural, to focus on the pain and misery of the situation and the circumstances rather than the gain, which is God's purpose in it.

Moreover, when the heat of life and bodily problems are there on a day-to-day basis, it is easy to lose focus upon a good God and His purpose. Yet, God is in the business of using what seems bad, for His glory and the believer's good.

Up to this point, I have presented three reasons why people – believers – don't emphasize that God's purpose in placing His people in union with Christ is to make them more like His Son. This truth is not preached from the pulpit, believers don't understand its significance if they have heard it, and believers are not convinced that God's purpose and design are best for them. I indicated that this results in a passivity by the believer and a turning from God's answers to contemporary wisdom. Sadly, I have witnessed this scenario as I care for my patients.

That brings us face to face with a crucial issue: Who is in control of this world and all that occurs in it? Further, the matter of control is brought home on a personal level when I ask individual patients: "Is God in control of what happens to you and your body? Has He made a mistake by placing you to have the body you have?" When I ask that question to a hurting patient, many believers falter. Why is that? That question, asked when no hard times are upon you, can be answered fairly easily – God is in control. However, when people and situations are not what you want, expect, hope for, or think you deserve, the heat and pressure of life force you to come to grips with your relationship to Christ. The crux of the matter, then, is summed by the question: What does your relationship with Christ mean in your daily life especially when you are hurting?

Patients' hopes and expectations collide with reality. Many different thoughts raised by this collision can be summarized by answers to following questions: Why isn't God giving me what I want? Is this really God's world? Does God have a right to run His world as He wants? Is God really good? Is God really powerful? Does He make mistakes?

These questions are not original and even echo the question posed by Rabbi Kushner in his book *Why Do Bad Things Happen To Good People?* Many agree with him that either God is not good but powerful or that He is good but not powerful. Either way, something is found wanting in God. These explanations are given in an attempt to help God out.

Apparently, Rabbi Kushner thinks that God needs his help and that God can't withstand the scrutiny of man's thinking. So in order to reconcile what God is doing with man's ideas, man chooses to recreate God in man's image. It is interesting that Rabbi Kushner (and others with his mindset) acknowledges God's sovereignty in bringing all things to pass.

What, then, is the problem? This thinking concludes that it is ungodly for God to cause, or even allow, bad things to happen to people – especially to me. It seems that Rabbi Kushner and others don't like His results and the way He brings things to pass. Why? They have defined "bad" using their own assumptions. "Bad" is something that they don't want, that they think they don't deserve, or that causes misery to them.

In contrast to human thinking is the truth of Scripture: God is God and He is not to be compared to any but Himself (Isaiah 40:18–28; 46:5–7). This is God's world and He runs it according to *His* wishes (Psalm 115:3; 135:6). He will not share His glory with another (Isaiah 42:8; 48:6–11). God has intent and purpose (Romans 8:28–29; Genesis 45:5ff.; 50:19–21). And this purpose is not only to demonstrate His own glory (Ephesians 1:11–12), but is also for the good of His people (Psalm 119:65–71; Isaiah 38:15–17; Romans 8:28–29).

Unless you come to grips with these truths, you will assume that God makes mistakes. You will assume that becoming more like Christ is not what it is "cracked up" to be, especially when compared to pain relief. You will assume that your relationship in Christ has little relevance to your daily life. You will assume that you must seek answers elsewhere.

Although patients may not say it in so many words, the thought of God's fallibility is often there. When asked if God has made a mistake, they express it this way: "I don't deserve this. I shouldn't have my pain and bodily problems." In essence, the patient is saying that his bodily problems and pain are evidence of God's mistake. It is as if He is saying that it was okay for God to do to Jesus what He did, but it is not okay for Him to bring this problem into the patient's life. This is tantamount to saying the patient deserves better treatment than God gave Jesus Christ.

Another misunderstanding is indicated by these comments: "God does not intend people to be sick – that includes me especially." Or consider this statement: "My faith is not able to make me well." This person has missed the point in two different ways: God doesn't need anyone's faith to bring about healing. It is not the person's faith but God's gift of faith, and more to the point, the God of that faith, Who brings about healing or nonhealing. God desires and expects faithfulness in the use of his gift (James 1:2-4, 5-8; 1 Peter 1:6-7).

After I tell patients about Romans 8:28–29, some, who don't like the situation they are in, comment on God's process of maturing faith in a less than favorable manner. These verses emphasize God's purpose in all things: changing and growing into Christlikeness. These patients will tell me: "I don't have time for this pain." "I don't see why I have to have this when I have tried so hard to do right." "I don't see how something so bad can be any good to me."

These statements accuse God of using means of growth that are unnecessary, insufficient, inadequate, not true, or at least "not for me." Therefore, that person's only recourse is to attempt to wrest control from God, muster up more faith (how much more?), seek after pain relief by whatever source he can, at whatever cost, and live in bondage. Why? His theology and view of God are wrong. God expects and equips believers to prove faithful. It is best for them and it glorifies God.

Some people, even if they are aware of the growing and changing principle, accept it as God's word, and are convinced it is good for them, are not sure how to apply this truth to their daily lives. They ask: "How do I use pain and bodily problems to grow and change when it hurts so?" "What does it mean to grow and change?" "Is there any way for me to know if I am growing and changing?" How do I examine and judge my inner-man activity? (2 Corinthians 13:5; Hebrews 3:12-13; 4:12.)

Let's begin by summarizing six Ps which focus the patient on God and what He is doing, rather than on his pain. Taking control of the mind (2 Corinthians 10:3–5, Philippians 4:8, 1 Peter 1:13) is the first step in getting victory daily when you hurt. In chapter 13, more will be said about specific "put-offs" and "put-ons" that flow from this changed thinking. The six Ps are:

1. God is *present*: He is in the problem. Therefore, the believer is not alone.

2. God has made *promises*: He is the true Promise Keeper. His word is trustworthy. He keeps His promises.

3. God is *powerful*: not only is God in the problem but He is active. He is not a God who sleeps.

4. God is *purposeful*: God wields His power, not in some arbitrary manner, but to accomplish His purpose – His glory and the good of each believer.

5. God is the *Provider*: He has made provisions to accomplish His purposes.

6. God is a *planner*: nothing takes God by surprise. He is not a reactive God. Rather, in eternity past, before the foundation of the world, God planned how best to glorify Himself for His Name's sake. In that plan all things are directed toward God's glory. The believer benefits because his good and God's glory are inseparably linked.

So, what is the believer to do? He commits himself to God daily. He focuses on who the Triune God is, what He has done in Christ, and what is doing by the Holy Spirit. How? He does this by relying on God's promises and His power to bring about what He has provided for in Christ. He recites God's promises and relies on God and His power. Words like "do," "commit," and "relying" are good ones but speak in general terms. We will explore how to apply the idea of these words to the problem of pain in the chapter 13. In this chapter, I want to be sure that you have a firm foundation by which to understand the truths presented throughout this book. Correct theology rightly applied produces right living. So if the essence of the Christian life is to be like Christ, then the Bible must have much to say about it.

Begin with Jesus. His relationship to and with His Father had significance for Him and for believers throughout the ages. His Father's teaching affected His life as the God-man. The Bible teaches that He was discipled by His Father in heaven and He did nothing on His own on earth (John 5:19–20, 30; 8:26; 12:49–50).

Jesus came to do His Father's will to accomplish a set purpose as the Triune God designed. Jesus' freedom was in living out that relationship by pleasing His Father and completing the work He was sent to do (John 4:31–34; see chapters 7, 9). He lived to please God because of His relationship with the Father. Pleasing God was in keeping with God's original design so it was Jesus' rule of life. His pursuit of that goal kept Him on track and His life was simplified. Jesus always kept the big picture and the end product in view.

That doesn't mean circumstances were to His liking, or that life was easy. Yet, Jesus was not focused on change of circumstances or pain relief but on living His earthly life in conformity to His Father's will. Consequently, Jesus had a satisfaction (even joy) about life because He wanted to please God. Jesus wanted to do His Father's will in place of His own (John 5:19–20, 30; 12:23–27).

Clearly Jesus is presented to be the Giver of abundant life (John 10:10–14). Believers are beckoned to keep their eyes fixed on Him Who is the Author and Perfector of their faith (Hebrews 12:1–3). The writer of Hebrews tells us why in these passages: Jesus was an "endurer" (v. 2).

And why was that? Because there was joy set before Him. What was that joy? It was a return to His rightful place of dignity and "Godness."

The believer's focus should be Jesus Himself (v. 3). If his focus is on Jesus, the promise is that the believer won't grow weary or give up (2 Corinthians 4:1, 16-18). Jesus didn't give up. Focusing on Jesus, what He did and how He did it, will help the believer model Jesus' focus on pleasing His Father. Enduring God's way for His honor enables the believer not simply to bear up under hard times but to gain victory in them.

What is enduring and bearing up? Bearing up under is not tolerating, coping, accepting, or getting by. On the contrary, the believer is never "under" the circumstances, for his God is the God of those circumstances. Rather, the believer focuses on using the circumstances as God intended – to grow. This is one lesson of the cross: using what is hard and hurtful to fulfill God's design.

What was good for the Father was good for Christ. What was good for Christ was good for the Father. Christ was exalted and so was the Father. What was good for the Son and the Father is good for the believer. God's glory and the believer's good are inextricably tied together. This is a crucial truth to call to mind (calling to mind is more than remembering) when faced with hard times, including pain and bodily problems. Calling to mind includes remembering: read, recite, and memorize. It moves further: it includes mediation on the truth, memorizing the truth, and actualizing the truth – putting it into practice (1 Peter 1:13-16). The believer is equipped by the Holy Spirit and so that he equips himself for competing the privilege of growing in Christlikeness.

Second, the Bible teaches that God's relationship to the believer not only began in Christ, but also is sustained through Christ. God began a work in believers and He expects a return on His work. He expects His stewards to give an account (Matthew 25:14–30; Luke 19:11–27; 1 Corinthians 4:1–5). He changed hearts, desires, and thoughts to enable believers to redefine life with all its problems from getting what they want, to doing what God wants (2 Corinthians 5:9, 14–15). Life is not spelled "relief" (see chapter 5). It is an opportunity to please God in thought, desire, and action thus following Jesus' example and command (Matthew 10:32-38; 16:23-24).

Consider this truth. God, the Creator and Re-Creator, is the One Who sent His Son to die a bloody, painful death as the holy, harmless, undefiled One in my place as my substitute accepting the penalty I rightly deserved for my sin and restoring my relationship with God (re-creation) through the presence and work of the Holy Spirit.

The believer ought to respond to this truth in at least four ways: thanksgiving (1 Thessalonians 5:18; Ephesians 5:20); testifying to God's greatness and glory by word and deed (Matthew 5:14–16); loving – showing compassion and forgiveness (Ephesians 4:32; Colossians 3:12–13); and considering it a privilege and blessing to serve, suffer, and evangelize (Philippians 1:29; 1 Peter 2:9–10, 21, 1 John 5:3-4).

Therefore, the believer can and should rejoice ("consider it pure joy") in various kinds of trials (and they will come!). In trials, his faith will be tested (James 1:2–4). To bring about the fulfillment of God's design, the believer's faith must be refined. When trials are handled God's way, endurance is the result. Faith is refined so that is it informed, intelligent, and active (James 2:14-26). The person shows himself faithful as his growth testifies to God's trustworthiness. The full effect of endurance is a completing of what is lacking – a more mature faith. "Maturing of faith" is another way of saying "becoming like Christ."

Trials, including pain itself or bodily problems, never make a person like Christ. They are the context for a believer's growth. Maturing faith can be defined as the development of Christlike characteristics and the fruit of the Spirit in any situation but especially in ties of discomfort and unpleasantness. Rather, responding to those tough situations by developing Christlike characteristics, including the fruit of the Spirit, is what maturing faith is about.

Endurance is necessary in producing mature faith. James does not say it is the pain that the believer is to rejoice in, but the effects that enduring will bring. It is not pain that is enjoyable, but the effects of pain rightly handled. Pain never causes spiritual growth; rather, using the pain as God's instruments to please God and to become more like Christ requires maturing faith.

It is easy, and almost reflexive, to groan and complain when hard times come. However, consider what happens when the believer thinks about his hard times as God's gift. It is easier for him to handle them God's way when he recognizes and appreciates them as sent by God to strengthen and complete his faith. Hope and endurance produce tangible results and feed on each other. Each enables the believer to use hard times to mature his faith. Moreover, each are the results of proper thinking and desiring about God, self, and the situation.

The Bible says that to please God, endurance is required (Romans 2:7). There is an active sense of the word, a steady persistence in well-doing, as well as a passive sense, bearing up under trials and difficulties. There is a tenacity associated with biblical endurance as we learn from Jacob (Genesis 32). Endurance is a characteristic of hope (Romans 5:1–5) so that without it, there is no endurance (1 Thessalonians 1:3). Endurance and hope are the key ingredients for long-term obedience. This triad always results in growing and changing.

Third, when pleasing God is the goal of life, the believer responds in a way that develops more of the character of Christ (Romans 8:28–29). And when he uses the daily discomfort and unpleasantness to become more like Christ, that is endurance. It brings forth a maturing of faith and strengthens a person's relationship with Christ (James 1:2–4).

Elsewhere, Paul speaks of believers actually boasting and being proud of what God in Christ has done for them, is doing for them through the Holy Spirit, and what He will do for them now and in future glory. Paul expects the believer to be excited about trouble. With hope and endurance, a believer is a winner undefeated by circumstances. The believer's God-given joy can never be taken away because of a body that he doesn't like. This is the best thing for the believer this side of heaven.

Biblical hope does much more. Consider what hope produces:

1. Patience as well as endurance (Romans 8:24–25; 2 Corinthians 4:16; 1 Thessalonians 1:3),

2. Confidence and boldness (2 Corinthians 3:12; Philippians 1:20),

3. Greater faith, love, and knowledge of the truth (Colossians 1:4–6; Titus 1:2),

4. Energy and enthusiasm with the ability to labor and work (1 Timothy 4:10),

5. Stability: hope is a safe and secure anchor (Hebrews 6:19) and

6. A more intimate and close relationship with God (Hebrews 7:19).

In taking care of patients, I find that they lack hope and, therefore, many do not endure or bear up under hard times. I find them (including believers) under the circumstances, burdened, and discouraged. I encourage them with the two Pss: patience and perseverance. Isaiah 40:29–31 summarizes these two Ps. In this passage, Isaiah points to Jehovah Himself as the Author and Giver of life (see also John 10:10–14). Those who hope (depend on, trust) in Him are "strengthened" (cf. Philippians 4:13) and, therefore, will not grow weary or faint. By way of contrast, Isaiah speaks of youths who grow tired, wear, and stumble in the midst of good or hard times. They do not have unlimited power. The vitality of youth is no match for those who Jehovah strengthens. Isaiah focused on God as the Giver of strength and endurance to those who hope in the Lord – those who seek to please Him rather to please self.

In 2 Corinthians 4:16-18, Paul writes that the fact of inner-man renewal is occurring daily while the outer man is decaying or perishing. The inner-man renewal is not automatic or instantaneous but continuous. Therefore believers don't give up. Decay of the body in its many forms is a given post-fall. Salvation does not reverse this decay. For the believer, inner-man renewal is an expected reality. It, too, is a given. These dual truths were an encouragement for Paul as he experienced and witnessed this renewal in himself and others.

Peter expresses this idea under the metaphor of fruit-bearing (2 Peter 1:3-9). In verse 4, he describes union with Christ (Paul's term for the relationship God establishes with believers) as participation or partaking in the divine nature. He urges believers who were wrongly treated by Rome to make every effort to grow their faith (see also 2 Peter 3:18). This exhortation is grounded in the promises of God Who is faithful and will never leave or forsake Christians. This God, Peter tells his readers, has given them everything they need to live life in a God-pleasing manner (2 Peter 1:3-4). These words are similar to Paul's recorded in

Ephesians 1:3 where he tells his readers that they have been "blessed with every spiritual blessing" in the heavens.

Fourth, the Bible calls believers not just "believers" or even "overcomers" and "victors" but something more. In Romans 8:35–37, Paul speaks of believers as "more than overcomers" or "more than victors." This reality is based on the believer's personal relationship with the personal, sovereign God Who causes "all things to work together for good." Paul spells out that "good": it is to be made into the image of Christ, to be like Jesus Christ (Romans 8:28–29). Then Paul refers to the love of Christ which Christ demonstrates to and for His people (Romans 8:35). This love is foundational and the reason why believers are and can be "more than conquerors."

Look at how it works. First in verse 35, Paul asks the question: "Who can separate us from the love of Christ?" He then lists any conceivable situation that a person might experience and all things that life can throw at you – and then some. This very impressive list includes "affliction (troubles in general), distress, persecution, famine, nakedness, danger and sword." These seven are general categories. You must fill in the specifics.

In verse 36, Paul, quoting from Psalm 44:22, says that these things lead us around as if we are sheep to be slaughtered. Paul is speaking of bondage and enslavement. Believers are pictured as putty in the hands of "things" and circumstances. But in verse 37, Paul makes clear what he is saying: No! What human thought and the appearance of things seem to indicate are not true for the believer when viewed from God's perspective.

Rather, in all of these things (not out of them!), believers are "more than conquerors" – "more than overcomers" through the One Who loved them. Christ is the Overcomer par excellence. Since He is the Overcomer, His people also can be and are more than conquerors by seeing hard times and situations as God sees them, and using them as God intended (v. 28–29). Go back to Paul's list in verse 35. People do respond to the things of which Paul speaks – situations and circumstances. People, like you, are neither machines nor robots. They have hopes, fears, expectations, and goals.

Here are some phrases I hear when patients come to the office with pain relief on their minds: "I am trying to cope" (coper); "I try to tolerate it" (tolerator); "I am trying and doing the best I can" (trier or best-I-can-doer); "I will just accept it" (acceptor); "I am getting by" (get-by-er); "I am trying to survive" (would-be survivor); "all I want is to be as normal as possible and feel better" (normal-as-possible-er or feel-better-er). In the face of these things, Paul asks (Romans 8:35): Are believers to be just copers, tolerators, try-ers, best-doers, acceptors, get-by-ers, survivors, or normal-as-possible-ers? "No," says Paul. Get this now: in all these things, the saints are "more than conquerors."

Get the picture: it is victory-plus! The believer's status and hope dope not change due to circumstances. Rather, the circumstances expose and demonstrate this status as more than a conqueror. For the believer who is more than a conqueror, victory is not spelled "relief." It is not spelled coping, tolerating, trying, doing the best, accepting, getting by, surviving, or getting as normal as possible. It is not even being a "conqueror." Rather, victory is being and acting as more than a conqueror.

Christ was the ultimate One Who is *more* than conqueror. Through His infinite love, He established a personal relationship with His people individually and collectively. Believers can't any more lose their relationship with Him than they can lose His love. Since all things were designed to be used by believers to become like Christ and to further God's purposes, believers are and are to function as conquerors par excellence. Believers are more than conquerors when they use all things as God designed. Believers are more than conquerors when they use hard times to become more like Christ and please the Father. Jesus used the way of the cross to please His Father thus becoming the ultimate Victor. His victory is the believer's in any and every situation.

Fifth, there is yet another way to describe the thinking and responding that comes from a victorious relationship with Christ. The victorious believer spells victory this way: he sees and accepts God's goodness in every situation. Based on the promises of God, he knows and acts upon the biblical truth that God is in the situation and He is up to something good. Further, he knows that this "something good" is good for him personally because it is God's purpose. God's activity in any situation is purposeful. That purpose is stated in Romans 8:29: to become more like Christ.

Victory is also responding to the illness, not as a burden and liability, but as a blessing, an asset to the patient's personal growth and ministry. Paul discusses this in Philippians 1:12 through 18. Paul knew certain facts: he was in a Roman prison and he was a prisoner. He had a choice to make regarding whose prisoner he was. After considering the facts, he concluded he was not a Roman prisoner but a prisoner of the Lord. Further, he was convinced and saw evidence of at least one purpose of his imprisonment: the advancement of the gospel. This advancement occurred through both his ministry and that of the saints in the Philippian church.

Peter discusses becoming like Christ in terms of the testing and approving of one's personal faith (1 Peter 1:6–8). The circumstances surrounding this epistle are rather remarkable. First, consider Peter. He had been quick to open his mouth, had spoken Satanic counsel (Matthew 16:22–23), and had denied his Savior three times (Matthew 26:33–35, 56, 69–75). But God chose him to write this epistle.

Second, consider his readers. This congregation was headed for, if not already in the midst of, terrible persecution. Yet Peter knew both from Godly teaching and his own personal experience that faith, which is more valuable than gold, must be proven genuine and sincere. This adds to our understanding of the maturing of a believer's faith. Clearly, Peter says that the individual's maturity is to the praise, glory, and honor of Jesus Christ. Again, we see God's glory and the believer's benefit being inextricably linked.

Peter knew that trials are one of God's ways of bringing about this growth. In 1 Peter 1:6, he tells his readers that should be glad and rejoice even though what they were experiencing was unpleasant and even dangerous. Jesus taught the principle in John 16:20-22. Apparently after the Holy Spirit came the apostles never forgot the lesson. The gladness comes not because of the trials but because God's purpose for trials is recognized and hard times are used to sharpen and to prove faith genuine. Genuine or approved faith is Christlike faith. Peter, knowing the purpose behind this approving process, goes on to say that their faith will be found to glorify Jesus. Peter warns believers not to focus their rejoicing solely over what trials and hard times may do for them (which is much). Rather, Peter tells them about a God-focus, teaching that a mature faith brings honor and glory to God.

What is the benefit to the believer who thinks about life with a God-focus and is not controlled by unpleasantness, discomfort, circumstances, pain, or his desire to get rid of them. He uses what he does not like to grow and change. This is victory because growing and changing in any situation occurs only by the provision of God's grace and life is simplified.

In fact, as further benefit, God's way takes less of the believer's time, attention, and energy than other ways. In 1 Timothy 4:7-8, Paul taught that growing and changing requires discipline. It requires knowledge of the believer's identity, his destiny, the way to it, and a plan and design for the believer to journey as a victor and gain the winner's crown. These truths help to simply the believer's life. His choices between pleasing self and pleasing God are narrowed. They help point the way so that God's goal is the believer's goal are attainable. The believer can always become more like Christ. This assurance is an encouragement, hope-engendering, and endurance producing.

Jesus Himself, as the God-man, had to experience what it meant to be human, yet He was without sin. He matured and the vehicles for His maturing included staying close to His Father's Word and as he experienced a myriad of hard times and trouble including the prospect of going to hell on the cross. (Luke 2:40–52; Hebrews 2:10; 5:8–9). Jesus was made perfect through suffering and He learned obedience from what He suffered. These verses from the book of Hebrews teach that Jesus identified with fallen humanity, learning what it was to please God when using His power to please Himself was so enticing. In this way He qualified Himself to be our faithful and great High Priest (Hebrews 4:14–16).

Obedience is something that can be learned. Suffering speaks of hard things experienced by Jesus. The passages reflect on the hard things and times that Jesus experienced. Suffering refers to those hard times and does not necessarily indicate a person's response to and in them. Jesus always responded biblically. Jesus was placed in situations and each time had to make a choice: to please God or self. In keeping with Hebrews 4:14-16, Jesus, in His humanness, identified with the tension of self-pleasing and God-pleasing as a the result of the fall, especially during hard times of varying degrees and varying kinds. All believers are called to please God, becoming like Christ in their thoughts, desires, and actions. Jesus was able to choose, and therefore please His Father, because He knew and loved His Father. He knew that His Father was powerful and good with good purposes. Proper knowledge of His Father and their relationship and the fullness of the Holy Spirit were necessary for Jesus to function as God's kind of Messiah. The believer requires knowledge and the Holy Spirit to follow in Christ's footsteps. The believer will never go Christ's cross but he is called to deny himself what he wants for the beauty of pleasing God.

Where we are at this point can be summed up by the phrase "the doctrine of two ways." This teaching runs throughout the Bible. We see it expressed in such contrasts as saved versus unsaved, lost versus found, good versus evil, the narrow road versus the wide road, and light versus darkness. In following this doctrine, I have set out two theologies: one approaches pain and bodily problems God's way and the other approaches pain and bodily problems from all other perspectives. In chapters 8, 9, and 10, I have spent time presenting God's truth as it applies to pain and bodily problems. You might say those chapters represent a theology of pain. The reason for this effort relates to the fact that correct theology leads to correct living.

ILLUSTRATIONS OF PEOPLE WHO HAVE HAD VICTORY: A LOOK AT THE BOOK OF *HEBREWS*

In His Word, God has provided for His people by joining believers to Himself in Christ. The Bible highlights and illumines the reality and beauty of relationships. First, the relationship within the Godhead involves harmony of purpose and function. This is seen clearly in the plan of salvation in which the Father plans (Romans 8:30; Ephesians 1:3–4), the Son accomplishes (John 3:16; Romans 5:6–10; 6:2–11; Ephesians 2:4–6; 5:1–2; Colossians 3:1–4), and the Holy Spirit applies Christ's work to God's people (John 3; Romans 5:5; 8:9–11, 14; Galatians 5:16–18; Ephesians 1:13–14; 5:18; 1 John 3:24; 4:13). In chapters 8 through 10, we have looked at biblical principles that emphasize the importance and outworking of that relationship. Now, it is time to look at other parts of Scripture to further see this relationship in action in the lives of the saints.

To begin, consider the book of Hebrews, in particular chapter 11. This is one of the best known chapters in the book. Why is it there? It serves as a source of encouragement and fits one of the main thrusts of the book. Included in the chapter are examples of faithful men and women who faithfully and courageously endured hard times. The chapter gives the reason why they were able to do so: in faithfulness, God joined Himself to His people by His gift of faith. Accordingly, because their God was trustworthy and a true Promisekeeper, they believed Him. The question to each believer then, as well as today, is: In the crucible of hard times, are you standing firm making sure your name is included in the list of faithful men and women? In addition, we are concerned about what Hebrews 11 has to say to us as we continue our study of pain.

First, look at the context of the book. There is evidence that the book of Hebrews was written before the destruction of Jerusalem that occurred around 70AD. It was addressed to Jewish converts who were familiar with the Old Testament. Times were not easy. These saints were undergoing hard times from nonphysical persecution to impending physical persecution. Because of these circumstances, apparently some of the saints were wondering whether they should remain in the Christian faith or return to Judaism. They were doubting their faith. But more, they were tempted to doubt the Giver of that faith and the Object of that faith. The threat of apostasy was a real concern for the pastor writer of this epistle.

Therefore, Hebrews is a book of exhortations. The saints are exhorted to remain faithful in "the last days," in a time marked by "I don't like" situations. A major for the writing of this letter was to keep the saints close to the Lord. Constantly, the writer pleads and exhorts his readers to remain faithful to the gospel message and not drift away (Hebrews 2:1; 3:12; 4:11; 6:11–12; 10:22–25; 12:25).

How does he do this? The book could be entitled the "Book of Better Things." The theme of the book is that Christ is superior and better than all other things. He says, "Jesus is better than" the prophets (1:1–3), the angels (1:4–14), Moses (3:1–6), Joshua (4:8–11), Aaron (4:14–5:5; 7:11–28; 9:1–15, 23–28), and Melchizedek (7:1–10). Writing under the influence of the Holy Spirit, the author sought to motivate the people by setting forth fundamental truths about Jesus Christ and by urging them to act upon these truths. Paul has the same message in Romans 6:11-13. The message is the same: because you are in Christ, think and act as you should daily, especially when God providentially brings tough times.

The writer, sounding like the author of Proverbs, strengthens his message by pointing out the folly and foolishness of returning to the former way of life (Hebrews 2, 6, 10). And yet the twist he gives has not only to do with the "badness" of falling away but also with the goodness of standing firm and enduring. Why? Because Christianity is much, much better than Judaism. And that is because Christ is much, much better than anyone and everything!

At this point, we pick up the author's exhortation at the middle of Hebrews 10. Beginning with verse 19, the writer reiterates his call for perseverance. He bases this exhortation on the confidence (assurance) that we have to enter the Most Holy Place, the very presence of God, by the blood of Christ. In the Old Testament, the people collectively through their representative, a privileged high priest, could enter the Most Holy Place. The high priest entered only once per year and after he made sacrifice for himself and the people (Leviticus 16). What was formerly closed under the old covenant is now open to all believers. Believers have entered representatively into the very presence of God since they are joined to Christ by faith, and therefore have access to God through Jesus Christ. The writer stresses the fact of the believer's new identity which is expressed in verse 22. This identity is not one of a sinner but of a person with an inner, sprinkled heart cleansed from a guilty and evil conscience and an outer, cleansed body washed with pure water. Again, as Paul does in Romans 6:1-13, the writer emphasizes what the believer is in Christ. In Romans 12:1-2, Paul calls the reader to get busy in applying to life and "I don't like" situations the significance of what it means to be in Christ. To the Jew, who had grown up with and on the Levitical system of animal sacrifices, a constantly changing priesthood, and man-made laws and traditions, such free access into God's presence was not only a privilege but also a marvel. How could he turn back to his former bondage?

In Hebrews 10:23, the writer repeats his exhortation to hold firmly to the hope that we confess because God is the faithful Promise Maker and Promise Keeper. In verses 24 and 25, the writer stresses corporate responsibility in holding firm and places the church as the agent and location for discipling. In verses 32 through 34, he reminds the saints of their past actions. They had stood their ground and had done just as the writer was now exhorting them to do. Why waste that previous effort, especially since they know how to endure hard times?

In the following verses of Hebrews 10 he connects all that he has been saying in previous chapters. This includes: encouraging them in their new identity and emphasizing the privileges that new identity provides them (v. 19–23); setting forth the church's responsibility in standing firm (v. 23–25); adding another facet of their God (in v. 23, God was presented as the faithful Promise Maker and Keeper): He is a consuming fire (v. 26–31); reminding them of their previous actions of standing firm (v. 32–34).

He further exhorts that they not throw away or lose their confidence, which carries a great reward (v. 35). The reward was one they had already experienced to some degree in their present life (v. 19–23; 32–34) but would experience fully in heaven. The writer is continuing his purpose of motivating his readers to faithfulness. He gives the "punch line" in verse 36: endurance leads to receiving God's promise. He states the same thought in Hebrews 12:14, where he says that without holiness, it is impossible to see God. He warns that non-endurers are not genuine, and therefore, have no place in God's presence. He concludes chapter 10 (v. 39) by reminding them that genuine believers will not shrink and draw back into destruction. Those who endure will be saved. With that, the stage is set for chapter 11.

Hebrews 11 contains examples of men and women acting faithfully who relied on a trustworthy God to keep His promises. Chapter 11 obviously follows chapter 10 and is in keeping with the author's main theme and purpose of the letter: to encourage and motivate the saints to remain firm and persevere in hard times. This was written to instruct, warn, and admonish believers. The situation contrasts with another part of the New Testament: 1 Corinthians 10:1-13 in which Paul cites examples of unfaithfulness. However, both passages serve the same function: encouraging the saints to "hold tightly" to Jesus rather than to follow the pattern of their forefathers. Paul unmasks unfaithfulness and equates it with testing God (v.9). Paul, as does the author of the book of Hebrews, concludes with a message of hope (v.13): There is no unique situation or circumstance for the believer; God's faithfulness ensures that He has not forgotten the believer; No situation is unbearable and thus none exceeds the believer's ability to respond in a God-pleasing manner, and thereby grow and change, to become more like Christ.

All situations will come to an end such that the believer cannot say, "I can't," as God always provides Himself as the way of escape. The message of hope is clear in both passages of Scripture – God is faithful, is ever present, and supplies His grace for His people in all situations.

What is the point of this list of positive examples in Hebrews 11? The writer begins in verse 1 with the nearest thing the Bible gives to a formal definition of faith. God has given the believer new eyes because he has given him a new heart – spiritual eyes. He is able to think God's thoughts and desire what God desires. What the believer could not see with his physical eyes – God's faithfulness – he sees with his spiritual eyes and knows it as certain and sure. Believers honor God by pleasing Him in hard and easy times.

Consequently, that which one hopes for and looks forward to is as if he has already received it. Faith enables the believer to accept, understand, and act upon all that God has promised. Faith views the unseen world as real, although the believer has never seen it or been there. In a sense, faith translates believers into the future, enabling them to view present day troubles and difficulties in light of the future (see Romans 8:18, 2 Corinthians 4:16–18, and 1 Peter 1:6–9). In his commentary on Hebrews, Jay Adams asks:

> But what do we see in each example that he gives? Clearly this: By faith, they all put the unseen world first. Things in this world, including safety and life itself, meant nothing in comparison to that toward which they were looking. None of them received the fulfillment of the promise for which they were waiting – the heavenly life with God. These people, who had nothing more than God's promises, were able to face all sorts of trials because they believed. They acted as though what they were promised were already present – so certain were they that God's Word would/could not fail. That, as the writer will say, is the crux of the matter; it is what faith is all about.[78]

Faith is what every believer has and needs, to successfully persevere. This future perspective and the reality of the unseen world brings a realism to life that enables the believer, in the midst of difficulties, to stand firm, to overcome, and to grow using an "I don't like" situation as God's instrument for that growth. As the chapter ends, verses 38 through 40 point out two characteristics of persevering saints: the world was not worthy of them (v. 38) and God gave them a good testimony as they had given testimony and witness to God's grace even though none had received what was promised (v. 39). God had something better in store for them. When the consummation comes, all of

God's saints (both individually and collectively) will receive what He has promised in full measure (v. 40). God has others, especially among the Gentiles, to bring into His kingdom. Until the last of His called ones are into the fold and brought to faith in Christ Jesus, all things will not be fully accomplished. Yet, until then, believers must live by faith, focusing on the unseen as present reality impacting their present lives (Colossians 3:1–3; Habakkuk 2:4).

In his first letter, John discusses the object of faith – hope as both a future and present reality. The hope of seeing God face to face was a marvel to John (1 John 3:1–3). It testified to God's love (v. 1), confirmed the believer's adoption (v. 1), set the believer apart from the unsaved world (v. 1), and was the foundation for the process of daily, progressive sanctification (v. 3). That same hopeful perspective is what enables you to overcome, while having a body that hurts and does not work as you would like it to.

In the next chapter, I look at specific portions of the book of Revelation. This book was written to people who would become martyrs, enduring a great deal of pain. Perhaps in times of pain and suffering, you will want to reread the book of Revelation and these comments to strengthen you in your pain.

The books of Hebrews and Revelation both depict real people in real situations that were terribly unpleasant. The message of both books is similar but tailored to meet each group of readers in their individual circumstances.

The book of Hebrews focuses on people who were tempted to turn back. Their situation was similar to that of some of the Israelites, who while wandering in the wilderness longed to return to Egypt. They thought things were better in Egypt than in the very presence of God (Numbers

11–21). Yet the writer of Hebrews holds out living the present life through the eyes of faith. This enabled these people to peer into the unseen world and catch a glimpse of a sovereign God, active and powerful, and yet personal. He is the One Who works all things for His glory and their good.

The book of Revelation extends this by allowing the reader to enter heaven, in all its bliss, using the medium of visions. There, the soon-to-be martyrs and the reader are introduced to what awaits God's faithful servants. What awaits them is eternal fellowship with the ultimate Victor, God Himself, Who rights all wrongs and avenges the death of His saints. This makes the believer a victor as well and is a further expression of Romans 8:35–39. John introduces his readers to the ultimate human experience of seeing God face to face.

As discussed earlier (in chapters 8–10), we experience the next best thing to seeing God face to face when we are joined to Christ (union with Christ). That union matures when we grow and change, becoming more like Him in Christlikeness. Paul posed a fundamental theological question that demands a Godhonoring answer: what is pain now in whatever form compared to the heavenly bliss that is to come (Romans 8:18; 2 Corinthians 4:17)?

HOPE AND ENCOURAGEMENT ON THE MARTYR TRAIL[a]

Unlike the author of Hebrews, the author of Revelation is known: he is John the apostle (Revelation 1:1–2, 4). The book describes hard times similar to those depicted in the book of Hebrews. However, now physical persecution was in view. Roman authorities were enforcing emperor worship and believers, who held Christ as King and Lord, were facing increasing hostilities.

---

a   A martyr theme pervades the book of Revelation. Martyrs and soon-to-be-martyrs, who are witnesses for Christ in their lives and deaths, are pictured as overcomers. Christ is pictured as the supreme martyr and ultimate overcomer.

John himself experienced these present realities. He was a fellow-sufferer, fellow-endurer, co-partner, and companion in these troubled times (Revelation 1:9). The Greek word for "suffering," *thlipsis*, can mean general hardship and trouble. John writes from Patmos to encourage individual believers who are soon to be martyrs in an increasingly persecuted church.

The book is a message of encouragement and exhortation to the churches of Asia Minor and individual believers in view of the present reality of impending persecution of the greatest magnitude. Satan is pictured as unleashing his fury, making a last great attempt to destroy Christ's infant church (Revelation 8–11 and 13–19, especially chapters 11 and 17). It is a clear message of the book that Satan's wrath will be intense, but only for a brief and limited time. Many would die ignominiously, but in the end, the soon-to-be martyrs would triumph as Christ, the supreme Martyr, had overcome.

John takes his people into heaven as the means of encouraging them in the face of this impending destruction. Not only were these soon-to-be martyrs, they were yet-to-be-avenged martyrs. The scenes in heaven are intended to show that their destiny is in the hands of Christ, the Overcomer and Holder of the destiny of every man. And He will bring His power and might in judgment, thus satisfying Himself as the Righteous Judge and avenging His martyrs.

God vindicates His suffering people by judging the one who persecutes His church and by establishing His new kingdom. A major focus of the book is overcoming. Jesus is better than, in part because He is the Victor and Overcomer. Believers are victors and overcomers because they are in Him and enjoy his fruit. As the Victor and Overcomer Jesus avenges the enemies of His Church who appear to be I control

(Hebrews 2:8-9). It is about avenging the enemies of His church, who appear to be in control of the world. The book details the blessings in store for those who endure God's way for God's glory in the midst of hard times. It is about what blessing is in store for His people who seem to be under control of those enemies. The book had application and significance for the people living during those times as well as for saints living on the other side of the destruction of Jerusalem in 70 A.D. The message is relevant for believers in all ages. Apparently, the Holy Spirit considered the happenings in John's time of such magnitude and significance that the only place John and his people could obtain a proper perspective, encouragement, and hope was in heaven. In no other book of the Bible (except The book of Daniel) does the Holy Spirit take His people into heaven in order for them to get a heavenly perspective of their immediate life and the reality of it. Throughout the Bible, this principle is clear: believers should live their present life from the perspective of eternity (Job; Psalm 73; Matthew 6:19–21; 13:44–46; 25:1–13, 14–30, 31–46; Colossians 3:1–3; 1 Peter 1:3–5; James 5:7–12). This makes all the difference during times of suffering and pain.

At the time the book of Revelation was written, persecuted Christians may well have been asking: "What kind of God do I have? Does He really care? Is He really in control? Is His control good?" Widespread persecution was breaking out with more to come. As precious in God's eyes as the death of His saints may be (Psalm 116:15), more was at stake than simply what the eye could see. John informs his readers (in the midst of their difficulties!) that the seeming imbalance of power was in fact not real. It just appeared that way (Hebrews 2:7–9). God's providential control over all that was happening was one of the book's encouraging messages to the suffering churches and suffering saints. As a result

God expected the churches and the saints to endure hard times and stand firm even unto death. Apparently many did! The same message applies in all ages.

In Revelation 4 and 5, John begins the prophetic portion of the book. Here John and his readers first encounter an overwhelming sight: the victorious God and the victorious Lamb-Lion receiving unceasing worship and praise. He gives his readers a glimpse of what faith enables a believer to do: to look behind the scenes at the unseen. In this case, John was able to put into proper perspective the realities of pain, suffering, power, and world dominion. John makes clear that the present, as well as the future, belong to no man, not even the emperor of Rome.

All things, including time and events, belong to God, the One sitting on the throne and to Christ, the Overcomer. He bears the marks of His suffering and death, but He is risen (chapter 19), alive, and well, having won a decisive victory at the cross. This victory was not only over Rome (chapter 17) but also over the real enemy, Satan (chapters 12, 20). He, the successful Redeemer, is the One Who was worthy to open the scroll of human destiny, bringing God's judgments upon His enemies to avenge His martyrs. These judgments are not accessible to the gaze of men. He is the One worthy to receive universal worship both from the seen and unseen world, just as God, Who sits on the throne, receives that worship. He is King of Kings and Lord of Lords. And His people reign with Him (Revelation 1:17–18; 5:10; 7:14–17; 21:1–5; 22:3–5, 13–14).

What an extraordinary glimpse into the very operation of God Himself! Life on the earth now took a different perspective for these soon-to-be martyrs! Armed with this perspective which was based on God's providential control of all things, His promise to right all wrongs and this incredible scene in the heavens, so many of these believers were able to face Nero's lions and burning stakes courageously. God strengthened them, and He used this book as His instrument to do so. Today, God uses His Word to enable His children to face pain and misery as they too contemplate the heavenly joys that await them.

But who are the people who will reign with Him? At least in part, if not the whole, these are martyrs and soon-to-be martyrs. Throughout the letter, John refers to those who have gone before as God's witnesses. The Greek word for witness comes over into English as *martyr*. The word has become a technical term for one who is killed because of his witness for Christ. What does a martyr do? He or she gives testimony by bearing witness, testifying to the truth of Jesus Christ. How does he do it? Most had the opportunity to gain their freedom and obtain earthly peace for themselves at the cost of renouncing their faith. This price is what the martyrs refused to pay. John himself, who witnessed by his life, had been exiled to the island of Patmos (Revelation 1:9).

John mentions Antipas, who had already given his life at Pergamum (Revelation 2:13–17). He witnessed by his death. This was, in part, the signaling of an ever-widening persecution that was about to come. John warned the churches at Smyrna and at Philadelphia of the impending trouble (Revelation 2:10; 3:10; the word *thlipsis* is used in 2:10 The word translated a common word in the New Testament indicating a crushing, pressing, squeezing from an outside pressure with or without a response by the person.). John urged the saints at Smyrna and Philadelphia to keep on proving faithful even to death because their reward, the crown of life, would be great (1 Corinthians 9:25; 2 Timothy 4:8; James 1:12; Revelation 2:7; 3:11).

The martyr theme continues throughout the book (6:9–11; 7:13–17; 12:11; 13:7–10; 14:12–13; 16:5–7; 17:6; 18:20, 24; 19:2–3; 20:4). It is clear that the cry is for judgment. Consider Revelation 6:9-11. Beginning with verse 9, the martyrs are singled out. These "souls under the altar" had been slain for God's Word and for their testimony. Their blood had been poured out, shed, flowing forth in sacrifice. These people were not silent. They addressed God as "Sovereign Lord," emphasizing His absolute power, but also addressed Him as "holy and true," stressing His goodness, trustworthiness, and reliability. These latter terms harken back to the Old Testament term *chesed* The word refers to God and is translated as loving kindness, trustworthiness, grace, and favor. The term has a major emphasis: God's covenantal relationship with His people and His faithfulness, loyalty, and promise-keeping in carrying out that relationship.[a] The martyrs knew their God. The martyrs were steadfast to the end. But they cried out to God for judgment.

The martyrs were bearing witness in heaven, as they had done on earth, that God is Lord and that He will right all wrongs. They knew the world is His, not theirs, and justice is a divine prerogative, not theirs. The prayers of the martyrs reminds us of Jesus' action on the cross when He entrusted Himself to the One who could judge justly and returned good for evil (1 Peter 2:22–23). John is clear that power is to be administered by God alone in conformity to His nature and the principles that He set forth in His Word. God's power is to be used to push His agenda, which in part is the reversal of the world's judgment on His people (2 Thessalonians 1:5–12). The reason for God's "delay" is

---

a   God motivates His people to action using the designation: "I will be your God and you will be my people" throughout the Old Testament, beginning with Abraham, the man of faith, who was called to step out in faith in the One, True, Living God and His promises (Genesis 12:1-4).

given in Revelation 6:11. After receiving the proper garments, they were told to rest until the full complement of God's people, their fellow slaves and brothers, had been completed. Their fellow martyrs would experience the same choices and results of those choices. More had to come into the fold before God's judgment would fall.

As the cross demonstrated, suffering was the road to glory. The final destruction of evil comes in God's time, which is sure and certain. God's longsuffering is not without a termination (Revelation 10:6–7). It is no less true for God's people, who are faced with all types of "I don't like" situations including pain and bodily problems. They have the same assurance.

In Revelation 7, we encounter a blissful sight: a multitude of martyrs clothed in white robes, washed in the blood of the Lamb, standing before the throne of God, serving the One sitting on the throne, Who has spread His tent over them (7:14–17). The number of martyrs has multiplied. These must include some who came out of the great persecution. God's power, justice, and faithfulness are the foundation of the hope for the believer-martyr as God brings many sons to glory. These saints had come out of the great tribulation (The word translated tribulation indicates trouble in general).

These people were pictured as overshadowed by God in all His glory. There was an intimacy of God with His people. They not only lived with, but were encircled by Him (His tent). That is a far cry from the fear of seeing God face to face and the fear of dying that unbelievers will know (Genesis 16:13; 32:30; Exodus 33:20, 23; Judges 6:22–23; 13:22). The Lamb, Who is the living water and bread of life, satisfies every desire so that perfect satisfaction is the result (Revelation 7:16). In verse 17, the Lamb is the Shepherd Who guides (Psalm 23). God wipes away every tear from their eyes (Revelation 21:4). John constantly pictures the heavenly bliss of the winner's crown as motivation for his people to remain faithful and steadfast. What applies to these saints of old also applies to believers today who overcome in any "I don't like" situation.

The book of Revelation is the textbook for overcoming, the overcomer, and God's means of overcoming. According to Revelation 12:11, the overcomer is the martyr. We find this triumphant message: the martyrs have overcome Satan by their testimony, not by themselves, but by the blood of the Lamb. The saints did not love their lives so much as to shrink back from death itself. In a real sense, the book of Revelation has a threefold message: devotion, allegiance, and loyalty by a proper focus on who they are and Who God is.

Overcoming involves a sense of duty, but it is more. There is something delightfully satisfying to living with an eternal perspective. This is what Christ did (John 4:31–34; 5:19–20, 30; 12:23–27) and is what believers are called to do (Matthew 10:32–39; 16:24–25; Mark 8:34–35; Luke 9:23–24; 14:26–27; John 12:25). God knows best for His people during these tumultuous and momentous times. The time was at hand (Revelation 1:3; 22:10) and "demanded" something drastic (Revelation 1:3; 22:10). John takes his soon-to-be martyrs into heaven in order to secure a heavenly perspective.

The word translated for overcome has other meanings such as victorious and prevail. The word is used primarily by John and is encountered in the final promises to every church mentioned in the book (Revelation 2:7, 11, 17, 26; 3:5, 12, 21). These final promises These final promises are intended to encourage steadfastness and victory. They all look forward to the eternal state which is described in chapters 21 and 22. In these two chapters, John's prophecy pictures the future coming, the

judgment, and the eternal state, which includes the final triumph of
the overcoming witnesses of Christ.

In Revelation 21:7, John uses covenantal language to bring home the
fulfillment of God's promises to the overcomers who are the martyrs
(12:11). They have an inheritance, God will be their God, and they will
be His people. The inheritance of all things includes those blessings
spelled out in chapter 15:2-4, and in chapters 21 and 22 (see footnote,
page 174). In Revelation 3:21, the promise to motivate endurance is
that of fellowship with Christ forever. The Overcomer has defeated
the enemy and offers His fellow overcomers a place of preeminence
eternally (Revelation 17:14). Victory in Jesus is one of the main themes
of overcoming in the book of Revelation.[77]

John also uses the term for victory/victor in his gospel and in the
epistles authored by him (John 16:33) and his epistles (1 John 2:13–14;
4:4; 5:4–5). It is of interest to note Jesus' use of this word in John 16:33.
There, Jesus said to his apostles that they would have trouble, but that
He had overcome the world. Jesus affirms His status as the Overcomer
and the Victor to His band of men facing unparalleled times in their
lives. He spoke these words the night before He died. Jesus was speaking of his earthly and heavenly victory that appear to almost everyone
as utter defeat. The world considered Jesus a loser. The apostles had
their own misgivings. What loomed before them was the seeming defat
of Jesus and the seeming victory of the evil one. It was in the upper
room the night before He died that Jesus prepared these men for what
was ahead. He held an advanced theology class (John 13–17). Never had
so much theology been presented in such a short time. However, this
was appropriate and fitting for the occasion.

In the same way, in the book of Revelation, John meets the people in tumultuous times. He teaches what is appropriate and fitting for the occasion. In this case, he moves his people into the heavenly realms by visions. The seriousness of the time as depicted in John 16 and the book of Revelation justified John's and Jesus' intense theological teaching. The Holy Spirit knew that proper biblical teaching was instrumental for its proper application and in overcoming. The times were serious and intense as trouble abounded both for Jesus' apostles' and John's soon-to-be martyrs. The magnitude of these impending physical persecutions would be enormous. Many would die in horrible ways. Therefore, the Holy Spirit, using John, took these soon-to-be martyrs into heaven. During hard times, it is important to be reminded of Christ, the Overcomer, the believer's relationship to Christ as a fellow overcomer, and the final eternal state.

In Revelation 13, John reminds his readers that God's people will be given over to the beast (Rome, the last representative of Gentile world dominion). The Old Testament captures the theme of Israel captivity and bondage to non-Israelites such as Egypt, Assyria, and Babylon. In the Bible, physical bondage is often a metaphor for spiritual bondage (Luke 4:18-22) Note in verses 5 through 7 that the phrase, "he [the beast] was given," is used four times (in the original language) in those three verses. This indicates the beast's subordinate position and Revelation expresses the truth and the reality that the beast is God's agent functioning only under divine permission. This same theme is seen in the book of Job (Job 1:6-12; 2:1-7).

In Revelation 13:8, John tells his readers that the beast has willing followers who are in opposition to God, and whose names are not written in the book of life. Therefore, they do not belong to the Lamb

Who was slain. John assures his readers that what really matters is God's sovereign control, power, and authority. If one's name has been written in the book of life then he has a place of security and will never forgotten or his name removed. John's point is clear: nothing in history (including the salvation of God's people) is an afterthought on God's part (Ephesians 1:4; 1 Peter 1:19–21). God's eternal purpose and decree are in view. John contrasts the eternal, unchangeable, fixed purpose of God with the short, fleeting, and changeable character and power of evil.

This thought is similar to Daniel 7, and Paul's thinking in Romans 8:18 and 2 Corinthians 4:16-18. In these verses Paul contrasts the present sufferings of believers with the heavenly bliss of being in the very presence of a glorious God. John tells his readers to accept the realities of life since they are from the hand of God. Who will bring about His justice, righting all wrongs (see Jeremiah's letter to the exiles in chapter 29 and Habakkuk 3). John exhorts, warns, and encourages his readers to acknowledge and act upon the fact that God is Sovereign over all of life. He knows that they will need endurance and faithfulness, which also come from the hand of God – via the instrument of the very book he is writing!

John has been striking a triumphant note. He has been encouraging his readers to live with a future, eternal perspective. He bases this on the kind of God the saints have: He is sovereign and exercises power and authority in a way that brings glory to Himself and benefit to His saints. He provides the steadfastness and faithfulness of the saints as part of His perfect and good will.

Beginning in Revelation 14:6, John reiterates a main theme: evil will not triumph and any earthly triumph is only short-lived. God's judgment is coming, but in His own good time. He calls each one to account since there will be eternal consequences for their actions (14:7–11). In those verses, John is preparing fellow sufferers for impending persecution by painting the picture of the suffering of the wicked. The persecutors will become the persecuted, by God Himself. The temptation for believers is to escape by renouncing their faith. John makes it clear that there is more to life than present realities viewed through physical eyes only. There are eternal consequences to choices made in this life. Both believers and unbelievers must contend with this reality.

In Revelation 14:12 and 13, John comments that an upward, future gaze requires endurance. And in response to that steadfastness and endurance, believers can expect a commendation similar to that which Jesus describes in Matthew 25 and Luke 19: "well done good and faithful servant"; "come and share your master's happiness." John writes: "'Blessed are the dead who die in the Lord from now on.' 'Yes,' says the Spirit, 'they will rest from their labor, for their deeds will follow them'" (Revelation 14:13).

In John's vision, God is praised as the Holy One because He has judged and His judgments are just (16:5, 7). God will avenge the deaths of his martyred saints by giving blood to drink to those who delighted in their deaths. John goes on to say (18:20, 24) that the heavenly hosts will rejoice that evil has been judged for the way Rome treated the martyrs (this addresses the prayer of the saints in 6:9–11). And the multitude of heavenly hosts, including the martyrs, respond to these happenings by rejoicing still further. They worship God by praising and thanking Him for His judgments and avenging the blood of His martyrs (19:1–3).

John makes his final reference to the martyr trail in Revelation 20:4-6, where he focuses attention on those who have suffered for Christ's sake. The consequences and results of actions here on earth are important to our discussion. The martyrs were now sitting on thrones; judgment had been given to them; and they reigned with Christ (Luke 22:28-30). Here is an amazing picture of eternal bliss. The saints were in the very presence of God Himself as His co-regents living on in eternity. These martyrs have not lost everything. To the contrary, they have gained everything for they have gained Christ forever!

In the book of Revelation, John emphasized God's sovereign control, His activity in human history, His personal activity in the lives of His saints, the divine prerogative of judgment, the power and authority of God to judge and judge justly, the fact that God will not be mocked, the troubles and suffering of the saints, the short-lived triumph of evil, and the martyrs' final destiny. He maintains that God has won a decisive victory over evil. John has emphasized the here and now. That is where his readers were and are. John has taken the truths that God is sovereign, powerful, almighty, and good and juxtaposed those truths to the fact that His people are oppressed. He concludes that the wicked can do no more than what God allows and that God judges justly. God will avenge His martyrs.

We are now ready to apply these truths. Ms. Patient, who we met in chapter 3, reappears in the next chapter. We will accompany her during a typical day of her life for the purpose of helping her apply biblical truths when feelings say otherwise.

CHAPTER ELEVEN

PUTTING IT ALL TOGETHER: PRACTICAL WAYS TO GET VICTORY IN THE MIDST OF PAIN

HAVING STUDIED AT LENGTH GOD'S answers to pain and bodily problems, how do you use these answers in dealing with pain? Titus 1:1 makes it clear that truth is essential to godly living:

> *Paul, a servant of God and an apostle of Jesus Christ for the faith of God's elect and the knowledge of the truth that leads to godliness.*

Applying God's truth in daily life should be the goal of every believer. This may be difficult, especially when the believer is hurting. Let's look in on Ms. Patient again and see how I help her to apply these truths. Ms. Patient is a typical person with any medical diagnosis and a body she doesn't like. I have already determined her diagnosis and I am now moving into the area of treatment.

First, I will present her initial office visit (of course, in an abbreviated form). Then, I will look at several of her return visits. Determining "where she is" and "meeting" her there are important matters. This comes about as I take time to gather information and know her as a person (see chapter 3). Ms. patient could just as easily approach her pastor for help (and may have!). The same principles that are presented to Ms. Patient are applicable in other settings by those interested in bringing God's truth for problem solving.

Ms. Patient tells me she wants me to help her. I ask her,

—What kind of help would you like?

—Help me get rid of this pain that I have had so long.

Ms. Patient has identified herself and given her agenda.

—What have you done about getting pain relief?

—I have gone to several physicians, taken medicines, prayed about it, had others pray for me, taken vitamins and herbs, exercised as best I could, and gone to physical therapy including water aerobics.

I want to find out from her the results of the pursuit of her desire for pain relief. What I expect to learn is what I usually learn from most patients: her pursuit has not provided her with what she wants.

—What have been the results of your efforts? What have you accomplished in your pursuit?

—I still hurt. That's why I'm coming to you. It's so hard to go on at times.

Ms. Patient has told me about the futility of her pursuit. I need to help her see and accept that futility. How will I do that?

—Have your efforts achieved relief?

—Maybe some relief but I still hurt.

—How much relief is enough for you?

—More than I have.

—What if it is not possible to change the body you have or get the pain relief you want?

—I don't want to think about that, but I guess I would just have to accept it.

—Tell me what you mean by "accepting it."

—Just living with it, going on day by day, trying to cope and
get things done.

At this point it is important for me to learn Ms. Patient's thinking.
The reason for learning about her thinking is to help her connect her
thinking, desires, and pain.

—Tell me what you are thinking when you are living like that.

—I am thinking that it is so hard to live this way. I wish this
pain would go away. I really want it to get better so I can
do things.

Ms. Patient has told me not only about her thinking but also her wanting.

—Tell me what happens to your pain when you are thinking
and wanting the way you do.

—Sometimes my pain doesn't change, but most of the time
I feel worse and hurt more.

—Then what happens?

—I get upset and frustrated, or sometimes I get discouraged
and depressed and just lie down on a couch or bed.

—Then what happens to your pain?

—It usually gets worse.

Ms. Patient is beginning to see the futility of her past efforts and
the bondage of her continued pursuit of pain relief. She came wanting
me to help her get relief and I now have an entry gate for doing that.
Most patients seek relief by what I call "medical maneuvers," including
medication, injections, even surgery, or a combination thereof. She
has told me that her response to her bodily problem produces more
pain, which is the opposite of what she is looking for and pursuing.

Some patients get a handle on what I am presenting very quickly. Others never do. Sometimes, for others, it takes time to acknowledge their futility and bondage. In order to help patients connect their thinking and pain, I give a pain journal with an assignment (see Appendix A, page 215). The patient is to record any new and increased pain, the circumstances, thinking and wanting, and the results in terms of more or less pain.

In addition, I ask them to make a list of the factors that aggravate pain and those that lessen pain. And I give them a number of "Pain Papers" I have written (see page 215). These papers contain core material useful to a proper understanding of pain, rheumatic conditions, and my approach to treatment. They are designed to move a patient's interest from his own relief to applying God's truth for pain and bodily problems.

Ms. Patient returns with the completed assignment. She is on her way to accepting the futility of her pursuit (it is not always that easy!). For that reason, she is willing to consider changing her hopes and expectations. I thank and encourage her for the completed work:

—What have you found out in doing the assignment?

—I can see that my attitude affects my pain level. I can make myself worse when I get upset and frustrated or when I have a pity party.

Up to this point it makes little difference whether Ms. Patient is a believer or not in terms of ministering to her. (I use the word "ministering" because I consider my practice of medicine an extension of my ministry in God's kingdom.) The principles that I have discussed with her, when applied, do bring about pain relief whether the patient is a believer or not. What are those principles?

Patients come to the office with an agenda and pursuit of
that agenda;

Patients think about themselves such that they have an identity. They think and live by what they think of themselves
and want for themselves;

Pain relief may not be obtainable;

There is futility, dissatisfaction, and bondage when one pursues pain relief as a major goal in life;

Considering the results of the pursuit of pain relief may be
helpful in changing that pursuit;

There is a connection between thinking, wanting, feeling,
and pain perception.

Now, in an effort to help her, I will attempt to move her to consider
a better way.

—Do you have a plan to change how you think and what
you want?

—When I hurt, I try to think about something else and get
busy doing something. Sometimes I pray to God.

Ms. Patient is experiencing the fact of her God-created duplex-being:
the inner man, outer man connection (see chapters 6 and 7). At this
point she has told me that she prays to God. She has given me another
opportunity to bring God's truth to bear on her situation. So I ask,

—What do you pray for?

—I pray for relief and healing.

—What has been God's answer?

—I guess, no.

—So where do you go from here? How have you responded
to His "no?"

—I keep praying for relief.

—And if it doesn't come?

With that question, I have taken Ms. Patient to the threshold that divides believers from nonbelievers regarding their response to pain. She has told me that her source and standard for satisfaction and contentment in her life is pain relief. If she is an unbeliever, Ms. Patient would have to "settle" for the inferior goal of the self-focus of pain relief. And she would not, nor could she, acknowledge the God of that "no" (she has neither the desire nor the ability). If Ms. Patient is a believer, she should be ready to hear what the far superior source of satisfaction and contentment in life is: pleasing God.

God's word does provide further resources to bring her to a proper understanding of pain and its role in her life.

—I may lie on the couch and depress myself, or take a nerve
   pill, or take pain medicine, or I will ask God for Him to use
   this pain for His glory.

—What is your purpose in doing any or all of those things?

—I guess to get relief. I guess I want God to give it to me.

In our discussion, I learned she is a believer and has accepted Jesus as her Lord and Savior. Also, she has mentioned that fact in her answers to the questions at the end of each "Pain Paper."

Therefore, I will ask her about Romans 8:28–29 during this visit, or I will give her an assignment I have developed to take home based on those verses (see Appendix B, page 217). She returns with that assignment completed.

—What did you include in your list of "all things"?

—All things include my bodily problems and pain.

—What is God's purpose in these things?

—I am not sure.

—What does verse 29 say?

—To make me more like Christ.

—What do you think that means in regard to your pain?

—I am not sure. I don't see how something that hurts and
feels so bad can be good.

At this point she is willing to use Scripture to address her problem. I have given hope along the way, and she knows I am interested in helping her. She also acknowledges that the hope I present to her is not mine. She describes herself as struggling. She means the tunnel is so long without light, the mountain is so high she can't get up, and the hole so deep she can't climb out. Here I need to do some teaching regarding God's original design for believers from eternity past, her relationship with Christ, and the result of that union which is to be more like Christ. Now I hope you can see the necessity of chapters 8, 9, and 10.

I will try to convince her that becoming more like Christ and pleasing God is far superior to pain relief and is satisfying, even joyful, even when pain relief doesn't come. How will I do that? I will remind her of her previous experience of pursuing pain relief. Not only has it been futile but it has also been counterproductive: the intensity of her pain has increased. Further, there is no guarantee in this fallen world that pain relief will come to anyone.

Further still, I will move beyond her experience and thinking and remind her of God's original design for her. It is to become like Christ, and when she does, she is becoming a becomer. Becoming more like Christ began at regeneration and continues until every believer is called home. It is best for the believer on this earth and it glorifies

God. She is no longer in bondage to her search for pain relief, and that is best for her.

The foremost biblical truth that should confront Ms. Patient is that there is a sovereign, good God in her life. At this point, she may be willing to say God is good, but not the pain. To get at that truth, I ask,

—Does God make mistakes?

—I don't think so. I guess I have never really thought about it though.

—Would you read Psalm 119:65–71 and tell me what it says about God?

> Do good to your servant according to your word, O Lord.
> Teach me knowledge and good judgment, for I believe in
> your commands. Before I was afflicted I went astray, but
> now I obey your word. You are good, and what you do
> is good; teach me your decrees. Though the arrogant
> have smeared me with lies, I keep your precepts with
> all my heart. Their hearts are callous and unfeeling, but
> I delight in your law. It was good for me to be afflicted
> so that I might learn your decrees.

—It says He is good and all that He does is good.

—If the Bible teaches that, are you willing to accept it as the truth?

—Yes.

—Even if you are hurting?

—Yes.

—Why, then, would this good God say "no" to pain relief?

—I don't know.

—Can you think of any Scripture we have studied together that might help answer that?

—You mean Romans 8:28 and 29, which says to make me more like Christ?

—That's it. What do you think?

—I read it and hear it, but tell me how pain can be something good?

Ms. Patient is being confronted with God's sovereign control and His purpose. The issue now is not her professed faith but her operative faith as she finds herself in hard times. And she has gone to the only reliable source to help her: God's Word. She is telling me about her epistemology – her source of truth (see chapters 3 and 7).

Not only that, she is coming to grips with the significance of her relationship with Christ for daily living. She is truly in trench warfare! She has moved beyond using God's "no" as a carte blanche invitation to use whatever approaches are available to get what she desires (this includes God Himself). She now is coming face to face with God's answer in and to hard times. What is that answer? It is for her to become like Christ. Not only that, she is beginning to address God's means of using what feels bad for the purpose of becoming more like Christ. The answer to her question, "How can something that feels so bad be something good?" is best answered by appealing to Jesus and the cross.

—In John 4:31–34, what did Jesus say His mission on earth was?

—It was to do His Father's will, which is to please His Father.

—Right. How did He do that?

—He went to the cross.

—Right again. I ask her: How did Jesus go to the cross? His relationship with the Father through the Holy Spirit sustained

Him. He made the Triune's goal His. He looked forward to heaven which enabled him to remain on the earth as the Victorious Messiah. He looked beyond the pain, which was great. For Jesus, there was not only physical pain but the expectation of the reality of being separated from His Father. Yet, what did He do? Hebrews 12:1–3 gives us the answer:

Therefore, since we are surrounded by such a great cloud of witnesses, let us throw off everything that hinders and the sin that so easily entangles, and let us run with perseverance, the race marked out for us. Let us fix our eyes on Jesus, the author and perfecter of our faith, who for the joy set before him endured the cross, scorning its shame, and sat down at the right hand of the throne of God. Consider him who endured such opposition from sinful men, so that you will not grow weary and lose heart.

He looked through the pain to the gain, which was plenty. He saw His glory, the Father's glory, and even the believers' "glory."

—Are you telling me that pain is good because of what it can produce in me?

—You are on the right track. It is not pain itself though. Pain is God's instrument, or tool, to stimulate you to use the hard times to become like Jesus. So when you use the pain to grow and change, becoming like Christ, you are doing what Jesus discussed in John 4:31-34 and what Paul talks about in Romans 8:28-29.

—Well, how do I use my pain for that? That seems so, well, unnatural.

—Right again. It is unnatural because we have formed habits
in how we respond to things we don't like.

After I have done some teaching on the "put-off" and "put-on" dynamic of biblical change (Ephesians 4:17–24), I am ready to answer her question.

—There are several ways to begin. Consider one way which is
found in applying Galatians 5:16–18, and 19–23. There Paul
speaks of the fruit of the Spirit. He tells us what they are
and encourages believers to demonstrate them in their lives.
In your case, God has you in a place where he expects you
to use the pain and bodily problems as stimuli to develop
those fruit in your life.

—I have never thought of that before.

—I appreciate your honesty. If this came easy, God would
not have needed to give us the Holy Spirit. God's way limits
your options and therefore makes life simpler. You know
where you are going (pleasing God) and how to get there
(using pain to become more Christlike). Here is an assignment. On a piece of paper, in the first column, write down
the fruit of the Spirit, prioritizing them from those most
lacking in your life, whether you are experiencing pain or
not. In the next column, the "put-off" column, record your
unbiblical thinking and wanting when you experience new
or increased pain. And in a third column, which is the "put-on" column, write out which fruit of the Spirit you did or
began to produce as you focused on using the pain as God's
instrument to become like Christ. You can use your Pain
Journal (see Appendix C, page 219) to help you.

Ms. Patient returns and her assignment is completed.

—How did your time go?

—I am better. I am not having as much pain. I have been able to read some of the things that we have been studying. It makes sense. I still hurt but I am getting things done, and if I don't, I use that time to pray and be thankful for what I have been able to do.

—What do you attribute this to?

—I have hope. I don't have to stop hurting to be able to accomplish something, especially pleasing God. When I do hurt, it is very different to sit down and ask myself, "What fruit of the Spirit is God wanting to produce?" I get busy doing that and find that I don't hurt as much or that getting relief is not as important as pleasing God.

—How about the fruit of the Spirit?

—It was amazing. Peace is something I didn't have. I always seemed upset, not happy or satisfied. I usually felt that way when I was hurting. I now see I didn't like being interrupted so I would get upset.

—Then what?

—I would get on the kids or even my husband. But when I was going to do that last week, I stopped and remembered what we were talking about in Romans 8:28 and 29. I pulled out my index card and read the verses. I remembered that God is good. It is hard to remember that when I hurt.

—What helped you remember God's goodness?

—I focused on the fact that He had a purpose for me in this pain. He wanted me to use the hurts to make me more like Jesus. And I did!

—Tell me about it!

—Instead of yelling at the kids, I asked them to wait a while, and then I got up and read their favorite book with them. Jesus didn't yell or get upset when He was hurting. He thought about others. My pain actually got a little better when I did.

Ms. Patient has come full circle. I have seen this scenario before. I have addressed her as a whole person. I have paid attention to her physical problems. She knows that I have her interest at stake and will use the best medical science I can. However, she also knows that I am not simply a "body mechanic." She is viewing herself, her situation, others, and most importantly God much differently than when she came to see me the first time.

How do I help her continue to think and respond this way? In my practice, it is not feasible for me to see patients such as Ms. Patient weekly in the office.[a] And I don't have to. There are ways to help her continue to grow. I have categorized these ways under the headings of stewardship of the mind and of the body. Let's look at some of those ways.

Begin with proper thinking and wanting. Often people speak of the mind and brain as synonymous. They are not. The brain refers to the body. There is no word translated in the original biblical texts as

---

a   I have set aside time in my office practice to minister to patients (and others) in at least two ways: (1) I discuss with patients their answers recorded in the "Pain Papers." This time may or may not be "office time"; (2) I actually counsel patients. These patients have demonstrated a concern and desire for applying God's truth to the problem of pain. This is never "office time" although it may be done in another room in the office.

brain. Brain is part of the physical aspect of man. Mind is often used as a close synonym for heart. Every person thinks, desires, and even acts in both the inner and outer man. He is a whole person. The Bible addresses man as a whole person. Only the believer bring his whole person – thoughts, desires, and actions in line with biblical truth. Since she has the mind of Christ, I want to saturate her with truth (Psalm 119:9-11; 1 Corinthians 2;16; 2 Corinthians 10:5) These facts are designed to lead to knowledge, which is truth applied. Otherwise, knowledge puffs up (1 Corinthians 8:1). The "Pain Papers" provide me with a way of doing that. Remember, those papers contain core material regarding various rheumatic problems. Moreover, they are designed to stimulate her thinking toward a spiritual interest in solving problems. Ms Patient has moved to where she is applying God's answers in her life. What does she need to continue in that growth?

Unless Ms. Patient sees and acts upon a good God behind all things in her life and understands that "all things" work for her good and God's glory, she will continue to deny God's truth and forsake God's joy. She will continue to metaphorically drown in her condition and continue as an unhappy camper. Her condition will be continued evidence that God is unfaithful. The key is seeing and acknowledging God's good and superior purpose in her life. She must daily continue to answer the questions: What is the Creator's design and purpose for me? What is the Creator's design and purpose for "all things" in my life? And close behind, she must develop a thankful spirit for God's providence and His good purpose in allowing her to be in her present situation, remembering that His purpose is far better for her than she can know (1 Thessalonians 5:18; Ephesians 5:20). It is not the pain she should be thankful but what God is doing in that pain. More precisely, it is her as she views herself and condition through God rather than God through herself and the situation. Developing thankfulness will take hard work, especially discipline (1 Timothy 4:7–8).

So I will have her write out the two questions found in the paragraph above on index cards. She is to look at those cards when tempted to focus on the pain rather than the gain. She is to pull them out at other times during the day, even when she isn't tempted to grumble and complain. She is then to answer each question specifically. The answer to the first question is "to become like Christ by using the pain to do so." The answer to the second is how she will do that in her particular situation.[a]

For instance, consider when she is experiencing pain. In the past, she has taken to the couch or bed seeking relief. Now, she pulls out her card and reads God's purpose for her in this situation. Rather than engage in a pity party, she now relies on God's grace to complete her personal responsibilities. In other words, she uses her whole person to honor God.

In order to help Ms Patient regularly answer the two questions given previously, I have introduced the "Focus Index Card." On it is the question, "Where is my focus: on the pain (hard times and misery) or the gain (becoming more like Christ)?" I will have her write out the above question on an index card and review it throughout the day. When she does, she is to check off that she has done so and write out the results of her focus. When she experiences pain, she is to pull out the card and answer that question. In other words, by focusing on the gain, she

---

a   See Appendix D, page 221. I can help her by having her replace one focus for another (using the focus card). It is best for her to use the pain itself to become like Christ. That in itself is a change in Ms. Patient's thinking. Remember, she wanted to know how something that feels so bad can be good. Here it is: using it to become like Christ – this is what she was designed from eternity past to do now.

forces herself into a dependent position before God. That is faith in action, and faith grows when it is exercised in that fashion. That is an occasion for great joy and thanksgiving!

The only satisfying answer for Ms. Patient that makes any sense in a world of misery is that God is making enemies into believers who are becomers (even overcomers). This is not "mind over matter" (or positive thinking) as defined by the culture. Rather, as discussed in chapter 3, Ms. Patient is changing her thinking and wanting, by the help of the Spirit and the Word, bringing it into conformity to Jesus Christ (Romans 13:14; Galatians 3:27; Philippians 2:5).

Moreover, I will have Ms. Patient begin her day – as soon as she awakens – with a personalized version of Psalm 118:24: "This is the day the Lord has made; I will rejoice and be glad in it." Ms. Patient is now beginning to begin her day with biblical truth. This is one way to break the cycle that Ms. Patient had developed. The cycle is very common. Patients tell me that "I go to bed with pain and wake up with it." "If it is not there in the morning, then I wonder when it will come." Pain, and more accurately her desire for pain relief, have taken center stage in her life. This focus of pain relief results in focusing on the misery and unpleasantness of the situation. It usually leads to the cycle of "pain begetting more pain."

Ms. Patient has been introduced to the truth that becoming more like Christ is the essence of her Christian life. God's purpose in bringing believers into His kingdom is to make them not only believers, but also becomers. In that way he is preparing them for fellowship with Him in heaven. As becomers, the believer has a foretaste of heaven on this earth. If Ms. Patient fails to accept and apply this fundamental truth to her daily life, she will consider pain and her body as burdens rather than as blessings. It is a loving, gracious God Who purposed to gather to Himself a people who are becomers. Therefore, I will have Ms. Patient set aside some part of each day to record her thinking about this truth – how it helped her grow and change that day by developing a fruit of the Spirit. I will have her bring back to me what she wrote.

Often, I will use Psalm 32:10 and Proverbs 13:15 in this endeavor.

Many are the woes of the wicked, but the Lord's unfailing love
surrounds the man who trusts in him (Psalm 32:10).
Good understanding wins favor, but the way of the unfaithful
is hard (Proverbs 13:15).

Both verses speak of futility and its results. Ms. Patient has expended energy, money, resources, and thought, attempting to reverse what may or may not be reversible. She didn't get relief but more problems. Further, her pursuit has hindered her capacity to expend energy and time on the chief goal of becoming more like Christ. She then was ready to accept the inferiority of her pursuit of pain relief. She concluded that there must be something better. For Ms. Patient, seeking pain relief replaced God's design. She would not admit it but she has been competing with God. Her motivation in pursuing pain relief has placed her at cross purposes with God. And God doesn't bless the competition. When there is an emphasis on pain relief rather than stewardship of the body, the focus of life is self-pleasing. Self-centeredness never leads to true satisfaction. Why? The answer is rather simple. God designed us to be God-pleasers, and when we are not in harmony with God's design for us then we are out of harmony with God Himself.

In contrast, when a person's emphasis is on becoming like Christ, the focus of life is to please God using both hard and good times as tools for doing so. This leads to satisfaction in life (the culture calls this "happiness"), daily progress in becoming like Christ, and (as a by-product) the potential for reduction of pain.

So, it was essential for me to challenge her thinking about pain relief. I did that by asking her: "Do you agree that your pursuit has resulted in futility, and do you accept that fact?" She acknowledged and eventually accepted the futility of her present hope to achieve what is usually unachievable. In her time set aside for daily devotion, I will have her reflect on that fact periodically as a motivation for her to continue and increase her commitment to use the pain for God's purpose which is her growth.

Second, a change in her wanting and thinking will be evident as she focuses on a sovereign, good God and His purpose. She does that the first thing in the morning as she reads her memory card of Psalm 118:24. Her focus on God's purpose of growing and changing to become like Christ will facilitate a further change in her wanting and thinking. Those two build on each other. This is the place that Romans 8:28-29, is so important and helpful.

I have found that most patients don't know Romans 8:28 and 29 as a personal truth for them in their present situation. So acknowledging the truth of Scripture is the first step. The truth that God is in the problem means Ms. Patient is not alone. Not only is God in the problem, He is also actively working. Ms. Patient is amazed that her God is actively working for her good by working for His glory.

Third, pursuing and developing the fruit of the Spirit is tangible evidence of her change in wanting and thinking. When Ms. Patient uses her body to please God even when it doesn't work as she would like, she is developing Christlikeness. Paul lists the fruit of the Spirit in Galatians 5:22–23 as love, joy, peace, patience, kindness, goodness, faithfulness, gentleness, and self-control. The Spirit's fruit in the life of a believer is one of the goals of changed living, is one evidence of changed living, and is the product of changed living. As mentioned previously, I ask patients to make three columns listing the fruit in order of priority for their lives in the first column, their thinking and doing that is opposite to that fruit in the second column, and how the specific fruit they are to "put-on" will look in their life. They can add a fourth column for the results of this "put-off/put-on" activity (see Appendix C, page 219).

One patient told me she lacked peace in her life. It was something she desperately wanted. She reported that her bodily problems kept her from that peace. Thus, she was determined to get pain relief so she could have peace. It was a struggle for her to see a good God with a good purpose when she hurt, and it was greater struggle for her to use that which she did not like (pain) to become like Christ. She failed (refused?) to accept the biblical fact that as a believer, she had peace with God through no effort of her own (Romans 5:1-10). I needed to correct her theology. I needed to teach her truth and help her apply that truth to her life. Again you can see the importance of chapters 8 through 10.

God's way for her to rejoice in His peace was the same as it was for Christ. The believer is a victor in Christ and because he is he will function as one. Ms. Patient was beginning to understand that using what was unpleasant to become like Christ is one goal of all believers. God's way was for her to rejoice in the peace she already had in Christ. This peace was secured at the cross (Romans 8:1). Joy is a byproduct of knowing and trusting that God is working all things for His glory and Ms. Patient's good. She was beginning to understand that her definition of good and God's was not the same. Becoming more like Christ had to become more important than it had been. Following God's design for all believers meant freedom for Ms. Patient. Exercise of that freedom would result in becoming more like Christ.

Consider the fruit love. The Bible tells us that love is giving to meet a need, no matter the cost, and with the right motive (John 3:16; Ephesians 5:2, 25; 1 Corinthians 13:3). Only believers can love as God requires (1 John 4:4:7–8, 19). That is one reason that God has poured the Holy Spirit into the believer's heart (Romans 5:5). And to appreciate His love to us and to develop this love, God will put individual believers, such as Ms. Patient, in situations where it is not easy to love. So Ms. Patient tells me she is not easy to live with when she is hurting. That is the time to call to mind God's superior goal of Christlikeness. With that goal as her focus, she will use the unpleasantness around her and maybe even in her to respond with the fruits of the Spirit, love being one of them. Paul is speaking of whole-person change. Not only that, loving means serving others by ministering to them as her physical condition allows (more will be said on this later). So Ms. Patient will record loving thoughts and acts in her journal when she is tempted not to do so. This record will serve as tangible evidence for her growth and thereby will serve as an encouragement to her and those around her.

There will be times throughout the day that she will not "feel" like fulfilling certain responsibilities. These include such things as taking care of the house, the checkbook, and her family, and even getting dressed in the morning. It is tempting for her to say, "my body won't let me do so" or "I hurt." If that is true, then both Paul and the Holy Spirit are wrong (see Romans 8:35–39; 2 Corinthians 12:7–10).

When Ms. Patient responds to the lack of pain relief by using the unpleasantness and discomfort as her stimuli to develop Christlikeness, she is growing. This reminds me of the patient (a believer) I cared for who said she wanted to stop smoking but "couldn't." She reported that she had tried everything. I had her approach the issue from the standpoint of stewardship. She agreed that she was not taking care of her body and thus dishonored God. The physical craving was very much of a burden to her. She did not want that desire so continued to smoke even though it was at reduced amount. She was determined to avoid any bad feelings. Feeling bad whether from the problems of the day and more accurately her response to them, or the bad feeling that came as she reduced her smoking was her main target to avoid. She used smoking as a tool to please herself by avoiding bad feelings. It was a failure. She began to understand that she was using a desire which was a demand to dishonor God. When she began to use the desire rather than to remove I or satisfy it, she began to get victory and eventually stopped smoking. Why? It was because she used the desire to smoke as a signal to focus on pleasing God. She decided it was better to feel bad and please God. That is victory.

I encourage patients who have pain, along the same lines. I will help Ms. Patient view pain as a signal to trust God and His control over her body. That focus forces her to rely on His grace so she can and will function responsibly. And it is a signal for her to be thankful for God's goodness when she is uncomfortable. This makes her more like Christ.

Fourth, I have helped Ms. Patient change her source and standard for satisfaction and contentment. The change involves replacing both the inferior goal of having a different body from "what I have now" and the inferior source and standard of pain relief apart from good stewardship of the body, which she uses to measure her satisfaction. The far superior goal of becoming more like Christ is always attainable.

What makes becoming like Christ superior? Most basic is the fact that it is God's goal for all believers. And because it is God's goal, it is best for the believer and is achievable. Moreover, it is delightfully satisfying even when pain relief doesn't come. No one can reverse the curse of sin in life, guarantee pain relief, or make it possible to have a body that he likes. When one approaches life to get things, especially pain relief and my "kind of body," he is being led by feelings and the "I wantsies." This means that he is living as a sensual being: his senses and their fulfillment control him. The desire is to see with the physical eye, hear with the physical ear, and touch or be touched by the physical hand. Satisfaction, the sensual person believes, comes from the feelings. Yet Christ says that what one sees with the eyes of faith are far superior to the senses (John 4:31-34). How can I help Ms. Patient see with the eyes of faith?

There are many examples in the Bible that detail believers acting in faith (see chapters 11 and 12). Biblical faith is faith in Christ and makes salvation a certainty because God Himself is the object of faith (Galatians 2:20). Knowledge is involved in faith and faith seeks to understand. But not only that, faithful people seek to obey. That triad of faith, knowledge, and obedience characterized Abraham's faith. The more he stepped out trusting, relying on, and depending upon God and His promises, the more faithful he became. His faith grew. Abraham grew.

Ms. Patient is in the same situation as Abraham. What was humanly impossible for Abraham and Sarah was possible for God. Ms. Patient has had days that she thought were insurmountable – there was no way out, let alone a way to victory. Ms. Patient had not been looking at the certainty of things. I gave many examples of that fact. She had pitted her wanting, feelings, and experiences against God's truth and promises. What a deadly trio are thoughts divorced from biblical truth, feelings, or experience. These as standard for living compete with the living and written Word. We have also seen in her life examples of her growing in grace and faith (2 Peter 3:18). At these times she is taking God at His Word and thinking and acting on His promises. She is doing this by using what she thought was bad (pain) for good – growing in Christlikeness. She has trusted God as a trustworthy God and she is becoming a more trusting person. This is living by the eyes of faith and as a suprasensual person.

Fifth, Ms. Patient must practice daily mind-renewal according to such truths as those expressed in 2 Corinthians 5:14–15; 2 Corinthians 10:4–5; and Ephesians 4:22–24. The goal is to move her from being a self-pleaser to becoming a God-pleaser. What is mind-renewal and how does it come about? What is inner-man renewal and how does it occur? Inner-man renewal is changed thinking and wanting. It is a daily activity. The person in all situations actively, cognitively, purposefully and willfully focuses on Who God is and what He has done. No matter the situation, Ms. Patient engages in changed thinking and wanting as she implements what she has been learning. Beginning here, when the pressure of life is low, prepares her for the storms and even the tidal waves of God's providence.

The results of this changed focus is a commitment to daily trust a sovereign, good God. The way to practice innerman includes, reading, reciting, memorizing, mediating on, verbalizing, and applying biblical truth as a blessing and privilege. This takes time, energy, and endurance. The purpose is to bring about a change in Ms. Patient's thinking and responding. Time must be scheduled for this and Ms. Patient must adhere to that schedule. Another source for reading is Jerry Bridges' book *Trusting God*.[77] It has been a good help for patients.

Another means of inner-man renewal involves daily reflection on the six "Ps" mentioned in chapter 10. I will have Ms. Patient write the six "Ps" in one column and, in the other, record how each enabled her to get victory that day. A sample would be:

God's PRESENCE (He is in the problem; Hebrews 13:5–6). Ms. Patient wrote: "I am not alone. Knowing God is actively pursuing His glory and my good is reassuring and gives me hope."

God's PROMISES (He is up to something now and eternally; (Deuteronomy 4:34). Ms. Patient wrote: "God is not a liar." He never promises anything He will not deliver. I can count on Him. Therefore, I don't have to count on people or circumstances to change."

God's POWER (He is up to something; Proverbs 21:1, 31). Ms. Patient wrote: "Knowing God is not impotent means I don't have to try to get control. I have done a poor job with my way. He is powerful and will use that power for me."

God's PURPOSE (He is up to something good; Romans 8:28–29; Genesis 50:19–21). Ms. Patient wrote: "Knowing this is God's purpose means nothing occurs in this life by chance or accident. Everything, including my pain and bodily problems, has a design by God."

God's PROVISION (He is up to providing both saving and enabling grace; Romans 5:5; 2 Corinthians 9:8). Ms. Patient wrote: "I am so glad that God has provided for me. That He gave me my salvation by grace is great, but to know He sustains me and enables me, not just to survive or get by but to be *more* than a conqueror, is something really wonderful." God's PLAN (He is up to doing work that He planned in eternity past; Ephesians 1:4, 2:10, 5:27). Ms Patient wrote: "To think that all of this was planned when only God existed is mind-boggling. It helps me think of God as a GREAT God."

Let's turn our attention to the second major category of stewardship: that of the body or outer man. It is important to get Ms. Patient moving. She has been tempted to shut down and avoid movement and activity as a way to reduce pain. She has given in to her feelings and either gotten angry or indulged herself in a pity party. The "pain avoidance" approach did not produce the desired results she wanted and actually worsened the situation. Her response as a "couch potato" and often as a an angry person has facilitated her downward spiral.

But where do I begin with her, especially when she is hurting and doesn't have much motivation or hope to do so? Teaching at this point is very important. Throughout her visit with me, I have taught her the physical aspects of her bodily problems. Most patients with chronic medical problems, from whatever cause, have as common features the deconditioning of their bodies and abnormal body mechanics. That combination results in inefficiency of the body with more energy expended. Various daily activities are usually more difficult. As I have said previously, I often talk to patients about their 1960 Ford body, the one they don't like, as they tell me about their "hoped-for" 2018 Ford body. I explain to them that the 1960 Ford has good miles left if they use it as an old Ford instead of a new 2018 Ford.

The point of the explanation is this: it usually takes more time to accomplish a task when one's body works inefficiently. I instructed Ms.

Patient to take this into account when she sets her daily schedule, allowing herself extra time for certain tasks. I encouraged her to become organized and a schedule-setter. I asked her to work up a schedule and bring it to me.

Another way to encourage Ms. Patient is to establish a functional capacity. A functional capacity is simply whatever activity one is willing and able to do. Determining Ms. Patient's functional capacity is based on the principles of good stewardship and is always correlated with a person's physical ability and capacity. Either I can help Ms. Patient determine a functional capacity or have her see a physical therapist. I simply have a person do certain activities that involve the activities of daily living (such as walking, standing, sitting, bending, and lifting). The patient will tell me about the ease of doing those things. From there, a program is developed that is designed to improve the person's functional ability and capacity. It will take regular attention to this program for maximum benefit. So I start where Ms. Patient can and is willing to start. No level of activity is too low. I determine her functional activity and capacity level and begin there. The adage "no pain, no gain" is a good one but must be modified depending on the person, his willingness to get moving, and his condition.

Next, I will have Ms. Patient list her individual responsibilities. I encourage patients to prioritize these responsibilities according to biblical principles (Ephesians 6:5-9; Colossians 3:18–25). Her list should include responsibilities that correlate with her physical ability and capacity. For instance, if she marks house cleaning as a responsibility, I must see how it fits her bodily problems and medical diagnosis. A person who has RA and desires to clean her house all in one day, may not be practicing good stewardship. She may need a readjustment of her priorities and how she accomplishes those tasks.

The next step in implementing this "get moving" program is to complete personal responsibilities no matter how the patient feels. A bodily physical exercise program is also included. No joint is better than the muscle and tendon (soft tissue) that move that joint. Improving the function of the soft tissue generally results in an increased functional ability. So any program that is regular and usually without weight being transferred across the joint is indicated. Bicycling, swimming, and walking, especially on a treadmill, are satisfactory. Let's use walking as an example. I will have Ms. Patient start at whatever level fits her and then build upward in terms of time spent walking and the speed of that walking.

There you have it. Ministering to the whole person is the key to getting victory in the midst of pain. I have attempted to bring together sound theology and practical living. I hope you can see the necessity for a firm foundation. That foundation must be grounded in biblical truth. As Ms. Patient discovered, God's answers are far superior to any other.

CHAPTER TWELVE

CONCLUDING REMARKS

IT IS TIME TO PUT the finishing touches on our subject of pain and the desire for pain relief. I closed the first chapter with a number of questions and a promise to answer them. It is time to review the results of that promise.

The facts and figures given in chapter 1 confirm the reality that many people are suffering from pain. The first questions posed were these: What should a person think and do in regard to the figures given in that chapter? How should he respond? Where should one turn for answers? In answering those questions, one exercises a choice which is influenced and even determined by his understanding of God and himself; his purpose for existing; and his final authority. I have labored long and hard to encourage people such as you to follow Isaiah's call: to the law and the testimony (Isaiah 8:20). Isaiah's call is to the Bible because it is where God's authoritative answers are found, including those that pertain to pain and bodily problems. It must be our only source for answering these questions. In chapter 2 I gave an abbreviated overview of the pain system for the purpose facilitating godly stewardship of the whole person. The complexity of the human body is something to behold and should lead to the proper application of the biblical principles of good stewardship.

In chapter 3, we took a look at the mindset of a pain sufferer who reports pain. We learned that people have been labeled and often think of themselves in certain categories. Based on a person's perception of himself (he gives himself an identity) and what he has, he devises a plan and agenda based on his hopes, desires, fears, and expectations. Often, a person wants and even demands pain relief. This desire takes center stage in his life. In fact, that desire all too often becomes the controlling force in his life. He is in bondage to it, and consequently, he is willing to turn to any solution that gives him what he wants. He is ripe for turning to cultural and contemporary wisdom for answers.

In chapters 4 through 7, we explored some of the answers of the medical community and the culture, both secular and Christian, that are offered to pain sufferers. Varying success rates for giving people the pain relief they want by any number of methods and maneuvers were mentioned, but we saw that in the end, the results were often continuing pain. The desire for pain relief (relief from the body and condition that one has) and a return to that which he had before only began a downward slide on a slippery slope: increasing frustration, hopelessness, pain, sense of futility, and dissatisfaction even with life itself.

It was at this point that biblical truth stepped up to the plate, so to speak, and began to deliver. Beginning in chapter 8 and continuing through chapter 13, the truth from God's Word was presented to shine forth as a breath of cool, fresh air on a hot, humid, summer day or like drops of a continuous, gentle rain in a dry, parched land. The Bible forces us to face the reality of grief, misery, and pain in the world in which we live. The issue is not pain or no pain, but how one will respond to it. The Bible teaches that believes have a new relationship initially established in eternity past and in God's timing because a reality in life on earth. The believer is in Christ and is indwelt by the Holy Spirit. The Holy Spirit initiates, maintains, and strengthens the relationship. The believer, then, is one who was designed by God to glorify Him by pleasing Him through becoming more like His Son. This means developing Christlikeness in whatever situation God places the believer. God may use the believer's own activity or inactivity as His agent to accomplish his plan. The believer is to use both "I like" situations and "I don't like" situations as God's tool and his vehicle for progressive sanctification. Both of these are occasions for changed thinking and wanting to be expressed as the believer honors God. What a relief! Pleasing God as an aim in life is something the believer can achieve daily whether he gets pain relief or not. This is delightfully satisfying. It also means that the believer doesn't have to chase the elusive and sometimes controlling desire of pain relief at whatever cost, which more often than not, leads to more pain and less satisfaction. Otherwise the believer will live by feelings as his guide. In fact, bad feelings (often described as fear, worry, depression, and angry) are expected and even predicted. As a result life is complicated and feelings are an easy target for therapeutic interventions.

Not only does the Bible have answers, but its answers are far superior to those that contemporary wisdom has to offer. To bring that point home, we looked at God's heroes of faith in Hebrews 11 and went with John into heaven itself in the book of Revelation. In both books, we encountered real people with real problems, some of which were bodily problems or potential bodily problems. It was clear that these saints of old were motivated by a future, forward look rather than a gaze fixed on the present, personal, temporal, finite, and created. In this life, they did not receive what God had promised, because as the writer of Hebrews tells us, God had something better for them. So it is with all believers. The key to getting victory in this life is in being a good steward of all of life, including opportunities that may arise from pain and bodily problems. Developing Christlikeness should not be limited to hard times. But hard times more than easy times remind of the cross and its cost, God's eternal plan, and the believer has I Christ by the Holy Spirit.

Lastly, chapter 13 lists practical ways of application of the biblical truths discussed. Questions designed to probe the level of the "I wantsies" were set out. Based on a person's answers, I moved him face to face with the issue of the significance of his relationship with Jesus Christ. A simple way to put it is this: Does my professed faith in the Lord Jesus Christ operate in my daily life when faced with pain and bodily problems? One can find out what his relationship with Christ means when God says "no" to his request for pain relief.

The time to develop a biblical perspective on pain and bodily problems is when God, in His providence, has given you a body that has not yet experienced the full extent of the curse of sin. Daily growing and changing, out of gratitude for what God in Christ has done for you, points you heavenward and enables you to endure and be victorious in hard times as well as good.

My prayer is that God will use this book in some way, large or small, to further His kingdom by growing individual believers such as you and me.

Appendix A

Pain Journal

Describe what is happening around you when pain begins or gets worse.

In evaluating those events, describe what were you thinking *before* you began to hurt and *at the time* you were hurting.

    a. If the events were *pleasant*, what made them pleasant?

    b. If the events were *unpleasant*, what made them unpleasant?

In the middle of those events, and as they continued, what did you *think*?

    – How did your pain change?

In the middle of those events and as they continued, what did you *want*?

    – How did your pain change?

APPENDIX B

ROMANS 8:28-29 AND 1 THESSALONIANS 5:18

8:28: *And we know that in all things God works for the good of those who love him who have been called according to his purpose.*
8:29: *For those God foreknew he also predestined to be conformed to the likeness of his Son that he might be the first born of many brothers.*

5:18: *give thanks in all things, for this is God's will for you in Christ Jesus.*

1. When Paul opens verse 28 with the phrase, "And we know," what does this phrase emphasize?
2. Who are the "we" in verse 28? Give two reasons for your answer (the answers are in the verse).
3. Who and what do they know?
4. What does Paul expect them to know about God and about themselves?
5. What are "all things" in verse 28?
6. Name specific "all things" in your life.
7. From verse 29, what is the good of "all things"?
8. From verse 29, what is God's purpose for "all things"?
   a. What is your role in "all things?"

b. What is the good that Paul describes?

c. How does this purpose fit 1 Thessalonians 5:18?

d. For what does Paul expect believers to give thanks for in "all things"?

9. What is your response to God's purpose of "all things"?

a. Give reasons for your answers.

b. What is really happening vertically?

c. What is your response to your response and God's control?

10. What will happen in your daily life if you agree with God and act upon the truth that "all things" are intended by God for you to use to become more like Christ?

11. Give specific examples of how knowing that the purpose of all things is good – to make you more like Christ – helps you in the midst of trouble.

a. The trouble is not the key.

b. Your response is the key which is based on your view of God, his design and purposes, and you.

c. Write specific ways you will use God's providence – the events in your life - to become more Christ in thought, desire, and action.

12. When you are tempted to please self, record specific ways that you used these verses to think, desire, and act in a way that pleases God.

13. Record your response to God's providence from am to pm. How does it fit the hymn It is well with my soul? How does it fit Christ's prayer in the Garden?

Appendix C

Fruit of the Holy Spirit Work Sheet

Fruit	Put-off	Put-on	Results
List fruit in order of priority, beginning with the ones most lacking in your life	List thoughts, desires, actions opposing that fruit.	List thoughts, desires, actions replacing items in "put-off" column.	Record the results in terms of your pain.
1.			
2.			
3.			
4.			
5.			
6.			
7.			
8.			
9.			

Appendix D

(These questions are to be written on a 4 x 6 index card)

What is God's general design and purpose for me in this life?

What is God's specific design and purpose for "all things" in my life right now?

Write out your situation. How is it part of God's "all things."

In what ways (be specific) am I using this present situation to become more like Christ?

PRAYER AND THE BELIEVER'S RESPONSE

Seeing patients daily in the office, I ask: "What do you do when you hurt?" Many times what is included in their responses is: "I prayed." Often patients include "I prayed to God" in their arsenal of pain responses. I will follow up with questions something like these: "What has been His answer?" and "How have you responded to it?" The patients' responses to these questions are reflections of their understanding of the Bible's teachings on prayer and their relationships with God. Let's look at several people in the Bible with bodily problems and their responses to God's answer.

Before we do that, it would do us well to ask: What is prayer? In a culture honed on self-exaltation and abounding in "healing ministries," how we answer that simple question will have far-reaching effects for daily living. So, what is prayer? Prayer is speaking to God. For each one of us, it is my communication to God and it is one way: me to God. It is not God speaking to me, for He has already spoken in Jesus, the Living Word, and in His written Word, the Bible.

The general word for prayer in the New Testament is *proseuche*. All other words for prayer refer to a specific aspect of prayer. Prayer may include confession and adoration; thanksgiving; and requests including petitions and supplications..

Next, we need to be clear about why we should pray and about what God's purpose is for us to pray. We should pray because we are commanded to do so (Matthew 6:6–13; 7:7; Luke 11:1–13; Ephesians 6:18–20; Philippians 4:6; 1 Thessalonians 5:17), because Jesus did so – regularly – and we are to be Christlike (Matthew 14:23; Mark 1:35; 6:46; Luke 5:16; John 17), and because it is a privilege to do so (Matthew 6:8; 7:11; Luke 11:13). Without prayer, there is no connection to God. God is connected to all His creatures but intimately and effectively to His children, believers. Prayer is God's vehicle for believers to demonstrate their dependence, trust, and acknowledgment of Who God is: the sovereign Ruler of His world, Who invites His people to come to Him. He hears all prayers at all times and responds to every prayer. His response may be "no," "yes," or "wait." Prayer is for the believer's benefit – not God's – and it brings glory to God.

Armed with the above truths, let's look at Paul. Paul followed Jesus' example – he was a praying man, and he prayed for himself in 2 Corinthians 12:7 through 10. I have referenced these verses in another context (chapters 7 and 9). Verses 7 and 8 teach two truths. First, bodily problems can occur to prevent believers from sinning. Here, in Paul's case, it was to prevent pride. Second, Paul had an interest in having his "thorn in the flesh" removed.[a] Most view the thorn as a physical malady such as his eye problem (Galatians 4:19). It is best to consider the problem and Paul's response to it as a whole-person problem In fact, Paul entreated or besought the Lord three times to remove this thorn. Jesus taught such persistence in prayer (Luke 18:1–8). Paul's persistence was an expression of his confidence in seeking God that was based on his relationship with the Father in Christ by the Holy Spirit. This contrasts persistence based on a wrong view of God and prayer – as if God is some cosmic vending machine who exists for me to get what I want and think important for me to have.

In 2 Corinthians 12:9, God answers Paul's request. Paul lived in an era of direct revelation from God. Not only did Paul speak to God, but

---

a   Some take the "thorn in the flesh" to be spiritual in character. In that view, the thorn (*skolops*) would pierce or puncture Paul's flesh but not his body (*sarx*: inner man's habits and patterns of thinking and acting developed when he was "out" of Christ and in Adam, the old man), which was his arrogance lingering from his previous way of life as a Pharisee and unbeliever (Philippians 3:3–6).

God spoke to him. Today, we have God's answer in His Word. What was His answer? "No." God then told him why: His "no" was because God's power is made manifest in the fertile ground of Paul's impotence. Paul had no control or power to remove this "thorn." If he had had a vote on the presence or absence of the "thorn," he would have voted for it to be removed. However, God thought and decreed otherwise.

The next verse records Paul's response to God's "no" and to His explanation. What Paul did defies natural, secular human thinking. He rejoiced in his "thorn"! Better, and more accurately, Paul rejoiced in the benefit of his "thorn." How could Paul respond in this way? Paul knew God – or rather he knew that he was known by God and knew God's purpose for his "thorn" (Galatians 4:9, Romans 8:28-29). Paul's response is a living out of Jesus' words in Matthew 5:3: "Blessed are the poor in spirit, for theirs is the kingdom of heaven." Jesus was speaking of Himself and called all believers to model Him.

God does say "no" to earnest biblical prayer. He knows what is best. God is wise and good. He is powerful and displays that power for His glory and the good of the believer. Paul was satisfied and even content having things God's way – it was best for him. God uses tough times to expose what our prayer life is all about. When the heat of life is on "cool," prayer doesn't really stretch us. However, when the heat of life is turned up to "hot," prayer takes on an entirely different perspective. God uses hard times to expose a believer's view of Himself and prayer.

Let's look at another incident in the life of Paul. In Philippians 2:25-30, we read of Paul's concern for Epaphroditus.

> *But I think it is necessary to send back to you Epaphroditus,*
> *my brother, fellow worker and fellow soldier, who is also your*
> *messenger, whom you sent to take care of my needs. For he*

longs for all of you and is distressed because you heard he was
ill. Indeed he was ill and almost died. But God had mercy on
him, and not on him only but also on me, to spare me sorrow
upon sorrow. Therefore I am all the more eager to send him, so
that when you see him again, you may be glad and I may have
less anxiety. Welcome him in the Lord with great joy, and honor
men like him, because he almost died for the work of Christ
risking his life to make up for the help you could not give me.

Here we find Paul speaking in glowing terms about Epaphroditus.
He speaks of him in relation to himself (Paul) and then to the church.
Epaphroditus became ill; we don't know the nature of the illness, but
we know he recovered. At least one question stands out: Why hadn't
Paul, by miracle and prayer, brought about his healing sooner? We
assume Paul prayed for his healing and that God heard his prayer.
What was God's answer? Ultimately, God's answer was "yes," but not
immediately and it was not through Paul as God's instrument.

Clearly, we learn that even during the apostolic era – truly a charis-
matic age – apostles could not perform miracles at their own discretion.
Their work had to be in conformity with God's will. God works on
His timetable. And prayer is no cure-all. It does not operate mechani-
cally, producing your desired results. Prayer, too, must follow God's
will and direction.

Let's turn to the Old Testament to find another, but slightly different, example of God's "yes" in answer to a prayer for healing. Consider
Hezekiah. We read his story in 2 Kings 18 through 20; 2 Chronicles
29 through 32; and in Isaiah 36 through 39. Hezekiah was king of the
southern kingdom and one of the few kings who compared favorably
to David (2 Kings 18:3, 5). As a result of the influence of Isaiah and Micah,

Hezekiah led the reformation in Judah. He removed the high places, smashed the sacred stones, cut down the Asherah poles, broke into pieces the bronze snake (2 Kings 18:4), reopened the temple (2 Chronicles 29:3), and cleaned up worship in Jerusalem (2 Chronicles 30:14). The reform occurred during times of unrest and an Assyrian threat.

The Bible records Hezekiah's illness in Isaiah 38, 2 Kings 20, and 2 Chronicles 32:24-26. In God's providence, he like Epaphroditus was at the point of death (2 Kings 20:1-2; 2 Chronicles 32:24-25; Isaiah 38:1-2). The prophet Isaiah confirmed what human reasoning and Hezekiah's own thoughts suggested: death was imminent. In each account, we are told that Hezekiah prayed, petitioning God, and received a miraculous healing. Not only did he receive healing of his bodily problem but also God delivered Jerusalem from the hands of the Assyrians and told why (2 Kings 20:6): "I will defend this city for my sake and for the sake of my servant David." God is a promise- (covenant) making and promise- (covenant) keeping God. God had not changed His mind. Rather, He had used circumstances brought about by His providence to bring Hezekiah to a point of total impotence. Hezekiah sought the Lord. God answered, and in this case, with a "yes."

Isaiah 38:10 through 20, records Hezekiah's hymn of thanksgiving. Our concern is verses 15-17:

> But what can I say? He has spoken to me and he himself has done this. I will walk humbly all my years because of this anguish of my soul. Lord, by such things men live; and my spirit finds life in them too. You restored me to health and let me live. Surely it was for my benefit that I suffered such anguish. In your love you kept me from the pit of destruction; you have put my sins behind your back.

Hezekiah moves from grief and lamentation (vv. 10–14) to considering how to praise God. He concludes that his only logical response is to walk humbly (the word means softly or slowly) all his years. Hezekiah is talking about changed thinking that leads to changed action. Also, he addresses God as Sovereign Lord in verse 16. He speaks of a physical renewal – his bodily powers and strength – but also a nonphysical renewal – a return to his life as king in its fullness, comparing favorably to David. Hezekiah is acknowledging that men live by God's gracious words and deeds.

Further, Hezekiah is acknowledging what Psalm 119:65 through 71, and Hebrews 12:5 through 11 teach. Hezekiah looks back on his experience and sees a purposeful God. He commends God for His purpose. He was not rejoicing in the anguish and suffering but in the benefit. The word translated "benefit" is *shalom,* which refers to wholeness, completeness, and prosperity. Without God's providential activity in his life, including his illness as well as his healing, Hezekiah would not be a whole person. He would not be a person growing and becoming like Jesus Christ.

Hezekiah's response to God's answer is similar in content to Paul's response that we studied earlier. Although God's answer was "yes" to Hezekiah and "no" to Paul, each believer responded out of his view of God as present, personal, powerful, and purposeful. They each rejoiced in God's answer because it was His answer, and each saw a good God with a good purpose behind His answer.

Yet one must be careful how he handles God's "yes" and he handles God's "no." Paul handled God's "no" properly. God was honored and Paul was strengthened. Hezekiah did not handle God's "yes" well. The Bible tells us that God added fifteen years to his life (2 Kings 20:6; Isaiah

38:5). Hezekiah was a poor steward of this time. In Isaiah 39:1, we read that envoys from Babylon came to Jerusalem. Hezekiah's response was to show these pagans everything in his house and the temple. He is confronted by Isaiah for his folly. Isaiah then pronounces Babylon as Jerusalem's conqueror and describes for the first time in the book of Isaiah the Babylonian captivity. This is not to say that Hezekiah's folly was the cause of the captivity. The captivity had been prophesied previously (Deuteronomy 28:64–67; 30:3). What we can say is that God expects a return on that which He gives us. In Hezekiah's case, it was physical healing and fifteen years of added life. As in Hezekiah's case, if we aren't good stewards, there are consequences for us and our children's children (Isaiah 39:7). In those words of Isaiah, Hezekiah's selfishness seems apparent as he is more pleased with the absence of consequences upon himself than the effects of his actions upon his children. In considering God's "yes," if we selfishly respond to God's giving us what we want, it may not be best for us. In looking back over Hezekiah's life, he would have had an unmarred record without those last fifteen years.

"PAIN PAPERS" INFORMATION

The "Pain Papers" came about because I was not helping hurting people by using the Medical Model approach to diagnosis and treatment The Medical Model assumes symptoms result from some physical abnormality that requires treatment. The Medical Model moves in the realm of the natural, physical, and material. He has no place for biblical spirituality a biblically-based anthropology. This fact, in itself, was something of a shock to me. I had spent much of my life depending on the validity of the medical approach.

I am a board-certified rheumatologist and author of a number of articles in the medical literature. I didn't fully recognize it at the time, but there was something lacking in my patient care. Patients continued to stream into my office under bondage to pain and the desire for some relief. At the time, I was growing in my understanding of the sufficiency and superiority of God's truth in dealing with problems, including pain.

Therefore, I began to put down ideas and present them to patients for their critique. That process went on for some time until the present final product. At present, there are eight papers, which are entitled: (1) Pain is a Problem; (2) Arthritis and Rheumatism; (3) Treatment of Rheumatic Conditions: An Overview; (4) Does Your Attitude Help You Deal with Your Pain? (5) The Connection Between Depression, Stress, and Pain; (6) What is the Best Way to Produce a Changed Attitude and Thinking; (7) Is There Anything Superior to Positive Thinking for Pain Relief? (8) Is Pain Relief All There Is?

At the end of each paper are three questions I ask patients to answer: What have you learned? How did it help? What changes do you think you need to make? These answers serve to gather data, help me gain involvement with the patient, and offer solid information on which to begin good stewardship principles. Therefore, I am able to introduce biblical truth in order to help patients get victory in their pain.

END NOTES

CHAPTER 1

1. G. H. Holman, "Chronic Nonmalignant Pain," Clinical Geriatrics (1997), 5:21–39.

2. D. L. Wagner, "Options for the Management of Chronic Pain," Internal Medicine (1997), pp. 57–71. B. Aghabeigi, "The Pathophysiology of Pain," British Dental Journal (1992), 173:91–97.

3. Donald W. Swanson, ed., *Mayo Clinic on Chronic Pain* (Rochester: Mayo Clinic, 1999), p. 1.

4. L. W. Moreland and E. W. St. Clair, "The Use of Analgesics in the Management of Pain in Rheumatic Diseases," Rheumatic Disease Clinics of North America (1999), 25:153–191.

5. M. A. Caudill, G. H. Holman, and D. Turk, "Effective Ways to Manage Chronic Pain," *Patient Care,* 1996, pp. 154–172. N. J. Marcus, *Freedom from Pain* (Fireside, Rockefeller Center, 1995), p. 22.

6. D. W. Swanson, op. cit., p. 1. "The Role of Nonprescription Analgesics in Treating Mild to Moderate Pain," in Clinical Management Conference Proceedings for the Primary Care Physician and Pharmacist (University of Minnesota, Office of Continuing Medical Education, Universal Program Number 031–000–99–060–H01).

7. D. G. Borenstein, "Chronic Low Back Pain," Rheumatic Disease Clinics of North America (1996), 22:439–456.

8. N. M. Hadler, "Low Back Pain," in Arthritis and Allied Conditions, Vol. 2, ed. W. J. Koopman, 13th ed. (Baltimore: Williams and Wilkens, 1997), p. 1821–1835. S. J. Lipson, "Low Back Pain," in A Textbook of Rheumatology, Vol. 1, eds. W. N. Kelley et al., 5th ed. (Philadelphia: W. B. Saunders, 1997), pp. 439–456.

9. K. K. Nakano, "Neck Pain," in A Textbook of Rheumatology, Vol. 1, eds. W. N. Kelley et al., 5th ed. (Philadelphia: W. B. Saunders, 1997), pp. 394–412. J. G. Hardin and J. T. Halla, "Cervical Spine Syndromes," in Arthritis and Allied Conditions, Vol. 2, ed. W. J. Koopman, 13th ed. (Baltimore: Williams and Wilkens, 1997), pp. 1803–1811.

10. N. E. Lane and F. Wolfe, Musculoskeletal Medicine Rheumatic Disease Clinics of North America, 1996, 23: xi–xiii.

11. Ibid.

12. J. E. Hamack and C. L. Loprinzi, "Use of Orally Administered Opioids for Cancer-Related Pain," Mayo Clinic Proceedings (1994), 69:384–390.

13. Caudill, op. cit., pp. 154–172. "Interdisciplinary Medicine," Management of Chronic Pain: Clinical Considerations in Patients with Cardiovascular and Renal Risks (1998), 3:1–8. N. Raskin, "Headache," in Harrison's Principles of Internal Medicine, Vol. 1, eds. A. Fauci et al., 14th ed. (New York: McGraw-Hill, 1998), pp. 68–72.

14. Ibid.

CHAPTER 2

15. D. W. Swanson, "Understanding Pain," in Mayo Clinic on Chronic Pain, ed. D. W. Swanson, (Rochester: Mayo Clinic, 1999), pp. 2–5. I appreciate this publication. I have utilized some of the infor-

mation in this chapter in order to present a simplified overview of the pain system.

CHAPTER 3

16. Lambert, the Sheepish Lion (Walt Disney Productions, 1952).

CHAPTER 4

17. B. A. Huyser and J. C. Parker, "Negative Affect and Pain in Arthritis," *Rheumatic Disease Clinics of North America* (1999), 25:105–121. L. B. Bradley and K. A. Alberts, "Psychological and Behavioral Approaches to Pain Management for Patients with Rheumatic Disease," *Rheumatic Disease Clinics of North America* (1999), 25:215–232.

18. Huyser, op. cit., pp. 107–109. Bradley, op. cit., pp. 215–217. H. Merskey, "Psychological Medicine, Pain, and Musculoskeletal Disorders," Rheumatic Disease Clinics of North America (1996), 22:623–637. J. I. Hudson and H. G. Pope, "The Relationship Between Fibromyalgia and Major Depressive Disorder," Rheumatic Disease Clinics of North America (1996), 22:285–303. L. M. Smedstad and M. H. Liang, "Psychosocial Management of Rheumatic Diseases," in *A Textbook of Rheumatology*, Vol. 1, eds. W. N. Kelley et al., 5th ed. (Philadelphia: W. B. Saunders, 1997), pp. 534–540.

19. G. H. William and R. G. Dluhy, "Diseases of the Adrenal Cortex," in *Harrison's Principles of Internal Medicine*, Vol. 2, eds. A. S. Fauci et al., 14th ed. (New York: McGraw-Hill, 1998), pp. 2035–2057. L. J. Crofford and K. L. Casey, "Central Modulation of Pain Perception," Rheumatic Disease Clinics of North America (1999), 25:1–14. J. C. Chikanza and A. B. Grossman, "Reciprocal Interactions Between the Neuroendocrine and Immune Systems During Inflammation," Rheumatic Disease Clinics of North America (2000), 26:693–711.

G. Neeck and L. J. Crofford, "Neuroendocrine Perturbations in Fibromyalgia and Chronic Fatigue Syndrome," Rheumatic Disease Clinics of North America (2000), 26:989–1002. D. E. Yocum, W. L. Castro, and M. Cornett, "Exercise, Education, and Behavioral Modification as Alternative Therapy for Pain and Stress in Rheumatic Disease," Rheumatic Disease Clinics of North America (2000), 26:145–159.

20. B. B. Lahey, "Stress and Health," in *Psychology: An Introduction*, ed. B. B. Lahey, 5th ed. (Madison: Brown and Benchmark, 1995), pp. 498–521.

21. See Endnote 18.

22. Chikanza, Grossman.

23. See Endnote 18.

24. Bradley, op. cit., pp. 217–218. Lahey.

25. D. W. Swanson, "Managing Life's Stresses," in *Mayo Clinic on Chronic Pain*, ed. D. W. Swanson (Rochester: Mayo Clinic, 1999), pp. 87–94.

CHAPTER 5

26. *Mayo Clinic on Chronic Pain*, ed. D. W. Swanson, 1st ed. (Rochester: Mayo Clinic, 1999), pp. 141–47. N. J. Marcus, ed., *Freedom from Pain* (New York: Fireside, 1999), pp. 31–45. M. O'Koon Moss, "Arthritis Today's 'You First' Challenge: Part One: It Is All About You," *Arthritis Today* (2001), 15:64–73.

27. Swanson, op. cit., p. 1.

28. Marcus, op. cit., pp. 25, 194.

29. "The Role of Nonprescription Analgesics in Treating Mild to Moderate Pain," in *Clinical Management Conference Proceedings for the Primary Care Physician and Pharmacist* (Uni-

versity of Minnesota: Health Learning Systems, 2000), p. 4. Swanson, op. cit., pp. 35–40.

30. Marcus, op. cit., pp. 68, 194.

31. Ibid., pp. 138–152.

32. Swanson, op. cit., pp. 2, 8.

33. Ibid., p. 41.

34. J. R. Rice and D. S. Pisetky, "Pain in the Rheumatic Diseases: Practical Aspects of Diagnosis and Treatment," Rheumatic Disease Clinics of North America (1999), 25:15–30.

35. Swanson, op. cit., p. 35.

36. Ibid., p. 35.

37. Marcus, op. cit., p. 139.

CHAPTER 6

38. R. S. Panush, "Complementary and Alternative Therapies for Rheumatic Diseases I," Rheumatic Disease Clinics of North America (1999), 25:xiii–xviii.

39. Ibid., p. xiii.

40. Ibid., p. xv.

41. R. L. Hatch, M. A. Burg, and D. S. Naberhaus, "The Spiritual Involvement and Beliefs Scale," The Journal of Family Practice, 46:476–486.

42. Ibid., p. 476.

43. D. D. McKee and J. N. Chappel, "Spirituality and Medical Practice," The Journal of Family Practice (1992), 35:201–208. M. D. Culver and M. J. Kell, "Working with Chronic Pain Patients: Spirituality a Part of the Treatment Protocol," The American Journal of Pain Management (1995), 5:55–61.

44. McKee, op. cit., p. 201.

45. B. B. Jones and K. F. Faull, "Arthritis – A Spiritual Journey," Arthritis Care and Research (1999), 12:367–368.

46. Ibid.

47. Ibid., p. 367.

48. Ibid.

49. Culver, op. cit., p. 59.

50. Ibid.

51. Culver, op. cit., p. 55.

52. Ibid.

53. R. P. Sloan et al., "Should Physicians Prescribe Religious Activities?" *The New England Journal of Medicine*. 25; 342; 1913–1916. [[[???]]]

54. Ibid.

55. Ibid.

56. Ibid.

57. Ibid.

58. Ibid.

59. S. G. Post, C. M. Puchalski, and D. B. Larson, "Physicians and Patient Spirituality: Professional Boundaries, Competency, and Ethics," Annals of Internal Medicine (2000), 132:578–583.

60. Ibid., pp. 579, 581.

61. L. Gunderson, "Faith and Healing," Annals of Internal Medicine (2000), 132:169–172. This author includes statements from a variety of authors such as Harold G. Koening, Dale A. Mathews, Richard Sloan, and Dana King.

62. Ibid., p. 172.

63. Ibid.

64. Sloan, op. cit., p. 1915.

65. L. Guterman, "Doctors, Don't Try to Heal Thy Patients with Religion, a Researcher Urges," The Chronicle of Higher Education, 30 June 2000, A19.

66. Sloan, op. cit., p. 1914.

67. J. E. Adams, "Counseling and Man's Basic Environment," *A Theology of Christian Counseling* (Grand Rapids: Zondervan, 1979), p. 45.

CHAPTER 7

68. R. P. Sloan et al., "Should Physicians Prescribe Religious Activities?" New England Journal of Medicine (2000), 25:1913–1916. L. Gundersen, "Faith and Healing," Annals of Internal Medicine (2000), 132:169–172. L. Guterman, "Doctors, Don't Try to Heal Thy Patients with Religion, a Researcher Urges," The Chronicle of Higher Education, 30 June 2000, A19.

69. D. D. McKee and J. N. Chappel, "Spirituality and Medical Practice," The Journal of Family Practice (1992), 35:201–208. M. D. Culver and M. J. Kell, "Working with Chronic Pain Patients: Spirituality as Part of the Treatment Protocol," American Journal of Pain Management (1995), 5:55–61. Gundersen, op. cit., pp. 169–170.

70. C. Van Til, *The Defense of the Faith*, 3rd ed. (Phillipsburg: Presbyterian and Reformed, 1967), pp. 7–9, 96–105.

71. J. E. Adams, "Counseling and Suffering," *A Theology of Christian Counseling* (Grand Rapids: Zondervan, 1979), pp. 271–275.

72. A. Sanford, *The Healing Light: the Art and Method of Spiritual Healing* (Macalester Park Shakopee, 1972), pp. 17–20.

73. E. Kubler-Ross, *On Death and Dying* (Collier Books, 1997).

74. J. Eareckson Tada and S. Estes, *When God Weeps* (Grand Rapids: Zondervan, 1997), pp. 124–125.

CHAPTER 9

75. J. E. Adams, *A Call to Discernment* (Eugene: Harvest House, 1987), p. 32.

CHAPTER 10

76. J. E. Adams, *Maintaining the Delicate Balance in Christian Living* (Woodruff, SC: Timeless Texts, 1998), pp. 21–26.

77. L. Morris, *The Revelation of St. John* (Grand Rapids: Tyndale New Testament Commentaries, Eerdmans, 1980), pp. 15-40.

CHAPTER 11

78. Jerry Bridges, *Trusting God*, 5th ed. (Colorado Springs: Navpres).

CHAPTER 12

79. J. E. Adams, *The Christian Counselor's Commentary: Hebrews, James, I and II Peter, Jude* (Woodruff, SC: Timeless Texts, 1996), p. 101.

For more information about
Dr. Jim Halla
&
Pain
please visit:

www.JimHalla.com
JimHalla@gmail.com
facebook.com/JimHalla

For more information about
AMBASSADOR INTERNATIONAL
please visit:

www.ambassador-international.com
@AmbassadorIntl
www.facebook.com/AmbassadorIntl

www.ingramcontent.com/pod-product-compliance
Lightning Source LLC
Chambersburg PA
CBHW062051270326
41931CB00013B/3024